Aspirin

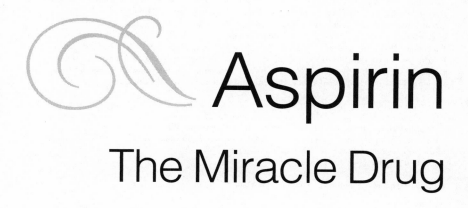

Aspirin
The Miracle Drug

Eric Metcalf

Avery
a member of
Penguin Group (USA) Inc.
New York

AVERY

Published by the Penguin Group
Penguin Group (USA) Inc., 375 Hudson Street, New York, New York 10014, USA • Penguin
Group (Canada), 10 Alcorn Avenue, Toronto, Ontario M4V 3B2, Canada (a division of Pearson
Penguin Canada Inc.) • Penguin Books Ltd, 80 Strand, London WC2R 0RL, England • Penguin
Ireland, 25 St Stephen's Green, Dublin 2, Ireland (a division of Penguin Books Ltd) • Penguin
Group (Australia), 250 Camberwell Road, Camberwell, Victoria 3124, Australia • (a division
of Pearson Australia Group Pty Ltd) • Penguin Books India Pvt Ltd, 11 Community Centre,
Panchsheel Park, New Delhi–110 017, India • Penguin Group (NZ), Cnr Airborne and Rosedale
Roads, Albany, Auckland 1310, New Zealand (a division of Pearson New Zealand Ltd) • Penguin
Books (South Africa) (Pty) Ltd, 24 Sturdee Avenue, Rosebank, Johannesburg 2196, South Africa
Penguin Books Ltd, Registered Offices: 80 Strand, London WC2R 0RL, England

Library of Congress Cataloging-in-Publication Data

Metcalf, Eric.
    Aspirin: the miracle drug / Eric Metcalf.
        p.   cm.
    Includes bibliographical references and index.
    ISBN 1-58333-218-9
        1. Aspirin—Popular works.   I. Title.
    RM666.A82M48   2005   2004062315
    615'783—dc22

Printed in the United States of America
10   9   8   7   6   5   4   3   2   1

Neither the author nor the publisher is engaged in rendering professional advice or services to the
individual reader. The ideas, procedures, and suggestions in this book are not intended as a substitute for consulting a physician. All matters regarding health require medical supervision. Neither
the author nor the publisher shall be liable or responsible for any loss, injury, or damage allegedly
arising from any information or suggestion in this book. The opinions expressed in this book repre-
sent the personal views of the author and not of the publisher.

Most Avery books are available at special quantity discounts for bulk purchase for sales promotions,
premiums, fund-raising, and educational needs. Special books or book excerpts also can be created
to fit specific needs. For details, write Penguin Group (USA) Inc. Special Markets, 375 Hudson
Street, New York, NY 10014.

While the author has made every effort to provide accurate telephone numbers and Internet ad-
dresses at the time of publication, neither the publisher nor the author assumes any responsibility
for errors, or for changes that occur after publication.

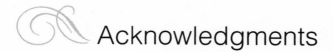 Acknowledgments

Thanks to Megan Newman, Scott Waxman, Farley Chase, Marilyn Allen, and M.V.A. for helping me onto—and through—this project.

Thanks to my family for their support, and, of course, to my wife, Laura, for doing far more than her share of caring for a newborn while I labored with this book.

Contents

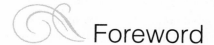 # Foreword

Aspirin is the grandfather and prototype drug of the family of medications known as nonsteroidal anti-inflammatory drugs (NSAIDs). Such drugs are widely used for their pain-relieving and anti-inflammatory ability, which makes them useful for controlling the discomfort and inflammation caused by headache, muscle cramps, premenstrual syndrome, and arthritis.

Although millions of people routinely take aspirin, ibuprofen, and other NSAIDs for control of pain and inflammation, observational studies show that these medications can also help prevent a variety of other serious medical conditions and chronic diseases.

In 1987, I personally began to conduct epidemiologic studies of aspirin, ibuprofen, and other NSAIDs, and their potential for the prevention of breast cancer, at the American Health Foundation in New York City. At that time, little work had been done to examine the association between cancer risk and sustained use of NSAIDs in human populations. I believed aberrant inflammation to be an important risk factor in cancer development, and hypothesized that agents with anti-inflammatory properties might reduce cancer risk. Our case control study, which took about five years to complete, clearly showed that sustained use of aspirin or ibuprofen significantly reduces the risk of breast cancer, and this helped set the stage for many other studies of NSAIDs and cancer. Since that first study, I have conducted and published the results of several additional epidemiologic studies. Most were at the Ohio State University Medical Center, showing that aspirin and other NSAIDs offer protection against breast cancer as well as other forms of malignancy such as prostate cancer and lung cancer.

A major breakthrough in our understanding of the benefits of aspirin came while researchers were studying prostaglandins and their health effects. Among other responsibilities these small "messenger molecules" trigger the immune system to react in response to viral and bacterial infection. (Prostaglandins are typically made by specific white blood cells of the immune system, but they can also be produced by other cells.) In 1992, researchers discovered another gene, cyclooxygenase-2 (COX-2), which controls production of prostaglandins.

Before the discovery of COX-2, scientists believed that the production of cyclooxygenase, which helps convert an essential fatty acid into prostaglandin molecules, was totally under the control of only one gene, cyclooxygenase-1 (COX-1). It is now known that COX-1 is a *housekeeping gene* that is always induced, or "turned on" and produces low levels of prostaglandins which protect various organs in the body, such as the lining of the stomach and the kidneys.

Conversely, COX-2, which is normally turned off, becomes turned on when there is an insult to the immune system such as a viral or bacterial infection, or exposure to a toxic chemical. The COX-2 gene therefore serves a very important function in the immune system: It provides the genetic signal in certain cells of the body, such as white blood cells, to begin production of prostaglandins, which in turn modulate the immune response to infection. Unfortunately, the COX-2 gene can be wrongly activated and become stuck in the ON position. As

Eric Metcalf points out in this book, scientific discovery has revealed that *the overexpression of COX-2 forms the basis of cancer development, atherosclerosis (the formation of plaque in arteries), and untoward inflammatory reactions in cells of the central nervous system.*

Aspirin and other NSAIDs that inhibit COX-2 are therefore profoundly important in reducing the risk of these debilitating and deadly conditions in humans. In recent years, the pharmaceutical industry has developed a new generation of NSAIDs called selective COX-2 inhibitors. Since these compounds (Vioxx, Celebrex, Mobic, Bextra) selectively block COX-2 without inhibiting COX-1, it was hoped that they would alleviate the pain and inflammation of arthritic conditions without increasing the risk of developing stomach ulcers or causing other adverse effects.

Unfortunately, one of these compounds, Vioxx, was recently recalled from the marketplace due to its potential for increasing the risk of cardiovascular disease in certain patients. Thus, while the selective COX-2 inhibitors are being reevaluated and newer compounds formulated for better safety and efficacy, now is a good time to remember that general NSAIDs such as aspirin and ibuprofen are still readily available over the counter and they relieve pain and prevent disease by blocking the same mechanism. Of course, any of these compounds should only be used judiciously, at low dosage, and under supervision of a physician.

Scientific investigations have found that regular, long-term use of aspirin and other NSAIDs significantly reduces the risk of a broad spectrum of diseases, including heart attack and stroke, most forms of cancer, and certain neurological conditions such as Alzheimer's disease. In this book, Eric Metcalf fluently captures the essence of these breakthrough discoveries that provide compelling proof that aspirin and related NSAIDs will ultimately have a significant role in the prevention and treatment of major life-threatening diseases.

Heightened prostaglandin biosynthesis can also produce genetic mutations and uncontrolled cell division leading to cancer in cells lining the colon, breasts, prostate, lungs, and other organs and tissues. For example, in breast tissue, activation of what is called the "prostaglandin cascade" results in heightened production of the hormone estrogen, raising a woman's risk of breast cancer. Inflammation due to prostaglandins also heightens the risk of developing Alzheimer's disease.

As mentioned, however, aspirin, ibuprofen, and other NSAIDs block the formation of prostaglandins by inhibiting the enzyme cyclooxygenase. By dampening this prostaglandin cascade, regular aspirin use can effectively reduce your risk of developing these life-threatening conditions.

Recent important scientific studies are documented in the pages of this book, revealing that use of aspirin or other NSAIDs will have profound preventive and therapeutic impact on cancer, heart disease, and mental illness. Indeed, the revelation that aspirin and aspirinlike compounds have notable disease-preventive activities has revolutionized medical research. The author provides a brilliant discussion of these exciting discoveries, complete with accurate scientific references. I believe the reader will find the book to be not only a fascinating story of scientific progress but also a reliable source of information about the use of aspirin and related compounds in the prevention of major diseases that afflict so many of us today.

Randall E. Harris, M.D., Ph.D.
The Ohio State University Medical Center, Columbus, Ohio
April 2005

Section I

The Story of Aspirin

Aspirin is such a familiar ingredient in our daily lives that it's hard to imagine a world without it. Since the drug is now more than one hundred years old, it's likely that your parents and grandparents never knew a time when the familiar tablets weren't found in medicine cabinets everywhere.

Aspirin is older than the state of Oklahoma. It was around when the Wright brothers took their historic flight. It predates other common objects of modern life like kids' crayons, crossword puzzles, tea bags, and Band-Aids.

For centuries before it was invented, mankind took chemicals found in nature that are similar to aspirin for their aches and fevers. Generations of scientists looked for a better version before finally discovering aspirin.

Until the early 1970s, just how aspirin worked remained a mystery. The discovery of what it was doing in the body won a Nobel Prize.

The following section will reveal the fascinating history of aspirin and provide a glimpse of how it's improving the world's health, one tablet at a time. You'll also learn how aspirin works in the body, with a similar action protecting you from maladies from headaches to heart attacks.

1

Aspirin's History and Future

In 1895, a young chemist named Felix Hoffmann headed into the library and laboratory to begin research for a new work assignment.

The twenty-nine-year-old worked in the small but growing pharmaceutical division of a German company that was better known for making coal tar–based dyes for clothing. Hoffmann had been working to develop new yellow dyes, but his supervisor asked him to turn his attention in a new direction. Hoffmann's task was to find a better version of a drug called salicylic acid.

The chemist was already familiar with this chemical: His father took it to relieve his arthritis pain, but was no longer able to tolerate its terrible taste and the stomach upset it caused. Hoffmann spent the next two years in research, including digging through scientific papers penned by previous scientists who had studied salicylic acid, before he finally came upon a way to improve it.

His father—or so the story goes—had begged Hoffmann to find a better remedy for his pain, and he became the first person to take the new and improved version of salicylic acid. Within just a few years, the rest of the world would be discovering its many uses, too.

Hoffmann was merely the latest to try to improve on a chemical that had fascinated doctors and folk healers for generations. Mankind had known for thousands of years that certain plants—such as willow, myrtle, and poplar—held the ability to ease their aches, pains, and fever. These plants contain an ingredient called *salicin,* which is part of a larger family of chemicals called *salicylates.*

By the Middle Ages, treatments made from plants containing salicylate were enormously popular as folk remedies for aches, pains, and sundry maladies all around the body.

In the mid 1700s, an English clergyman named Reverend Edward Stone—whose varied interests included astronomy and medicine—began investigating the medical properties of willow bark. Europeans of the day were fond of using the bark of the cinchona tree of South America to treat fevers, which were sometimes caused by malaria. They were on the right track, since cinchona bark contains quinine, which is still used as a drug to treat malaria to this day.

Unfortunately, the trees couldn't be cultivated in Europe, and supplies of the bark were growing scarce due to the expense and difficulty of transporting it to Europe. Stone set about to find a substitute. He noted that the bitter taste of white willow bark reminded him of the flavor of the cinchona bark. Willow also looked promising because of the types of environment the trees preferred.

At the time, a prevailing medical theory called "The Doctrine of Signatures" held that the cure for a disease could often be found near its cause. Since fevers were thought to be more common in soggy environments, Stone

Beech and birch trees also contain salicylates, and so do tea, coffee, licorice, olives, wintergreen, strawberries, cherries, plums, oranges, and apples. Beavers secrete salicylates, too.

The Aspirin Vocabulary

- *Acetylsalicylic acid (ASA).* The chemical name of aspirin, a compound made by adding a molecule from a chemical relative of acetic acid (better known as vinegar) to salicylic acid.
- *Salicylates.* A group of similar chemicals that includes salicin and salicylic acid.
- *Salicylic acid.* Salicin turns into this in the body when consumed. Salicin can also be converted into salicylic acid in the laboratory. This is a main component in aspirin.
- *Salicin.* A chemical found in willow and poplar trees; it's the active ingredient that gives the plants their medicinal properties.

thought the white willow tree, which thrives in marshy areas, would be a good candidate as a treatment for this condition.

He dried a quantity of bark outside a baker's oven for three months, and over the course of the next few years he gave dried, pulverized willow bark to more than fifty patients suffering from fevers and stiffness. He found that the remedy worked with great success in curing his test subjects' ills, and he reported his results in a paper to the Royal Society of London in 1763.

By the mid-1800s, a number of researchers had begun laboring to pinpoint just what ingredient was lurking in willow that made it such a useful herbal medicine, and then manipulating the chemical to make it work better. In 1829 a French pharmacist by the name of Henri Leroux isolated the bitter salicin from willow bark. When people consume willow bark, the salicin is converted into salicylic acid in the body. A chemist can also derive salicylic acid from salicin in the laboratory, which researchers learned to do in the 1830s.

Salicylic acid also became used as an antiseptic in surgeries—and as a preservative for milk, beer, and other foods.

Physicians throughout the century issued research papers that detailed their success in using salicin and salicylic acid to treat rheumatic fever, gout, and the fever caused by typhoid.

In 1853 a French chemist named Charles von Gerhardt created a crude, synthetic version of salicylic acid called acetylsalicylic acid (ASA). No one paid much attention to his discovery at the time. Decades later, though, Gerhardt's work caught the eye of Felix Hoffmann the chemist.

Aspirin-like Chemicals Keep *Plants* Healthy, Too

Aspirin can work wonders throughout your body, as you'll learn in this book. But the chemicals similar to aspirin found naturally in plants work in amazing ways to keep *them* healthy, too.

Most plants—perhaps all of them—produce traces of chemicals called salicylates.

When plants are under attack, like from bacteria, fungi, and insects, these tiny amounts of salicylates take part in a cascade of chemical responses within the plant. This defensive activity may cause the plant to produce enzymes or toxins that harm the attacker, says Don Cipollini, Ph.D., an associate professor in the department of biological sciences at Wright State University in Dayton.

"Plants have to sit there and take whatever comes their way. They can't get up and run away, and they can't shake off an insect. So they have to shake it off chemically," he says. In this regard, the salicylates act similarly to hormones in humans by relaying messages chemically throughout the plant. And similar to humans' immune system, the plant can relay these chemical signals to other leaves that aren't yet under attack, to help *them* resist later attacks, too.

The salicylates may also help plants regulate their temperature, allowing them to tolerate heat and cold better, he says. This is particularly interesting when you take into account that aspirin reduces fever in humans.

Some plants produce more than just traces of salicylate; some, like the willow, poplar, and aspen trees, produce it in high concentrations. In these plants, the larger concentration of chemicals can directly injure creatures that eat them, says Rick Lindroth, Ph.D., a University of Wisconsin professor who studies interactions between plants and insects.

If a bug isn't accustomed to eating these plants, or it gobbles down a particular leaf with an extra-high concentration of salicylate, the plant can cause the insect's guts to break down, leading to death. Again, there's a connection to humans there, since too much aspirin can give you stomach and intestinal damage.

Gypsy moths, however, are accustomed to chewing on aspen trees, in which salicylates may account for 10 percent of their dry weight. The average gypsy moth eats enough salicylate each day to equal a 150-pound person swallowing about *6 pounds* of aspirin daily, which would certainly spell hasty doom for a human.

Ever seen a gypsy moth with a headache? Didn't think so.

While Hoffmann was combing through the scientific literature during his research to find a version of salicylic acid that didn't cause vomiting—a common side effect—he realized that Gerhardt was onto something. Hoffman devised a way to improve upon Gerhardt's method of creating ASA by chemically combining salicylic acid with acetic acid, which in diluted form is better known as vinegar.

Aspirin today is still made with a chemical relative of vinegar, and bottles of aspirin that have been sitting around your house for too long will have the familiar pungent odor. That's a sign that you need to toss them and buy fresh aspirin. In Hoffman's day, the salicylic acid came from coal tar, and nowadays it usually comes from petroleum, thus sparing forests of willow trees.

Hoffmann hoped that *acetylizing* the salicylic acid—which means to add a molecule called an acetyl group to the salicylic acid's structure—would make the chemical gentler on the stomach and allow the body to absorb it better.

But he could have no way of knowing at the time that this addition to the salicylic acid would also give the drug a remarkable ability to treat and prevent many serious and deadly diseases.

Hoffmann's father reportedly found that ASA relieved his arthritis pain without causing stomach upset like salicylic acid did. Hoffmann's supervisors, however, weren't particularly interested in further developing ASA at first, for reasons we'll get to in chapter 3. But they eventually realized its potential and decided to bring it to the public.

The company's chief pharmacologist decided to call the drug "Aspirin." He came about the name by taking the word *Spiraea*—the name for the genus of plants that contains meadowsweet, which contains a salicylate—and adding an "a" at the front, which stood for the acetylation process. However, some claim that the drug is named for Saint Aspirinius, an early bishop who was the patron saint of . . . headaches.

The German company patented the name and the process for making the drug in 1899, and Aspirin spread quickly around the world, where it would soon become the most widely used drug on the planet. That's Aspirin with a capital A, mind you; only this single company made the drug, and it was all theirs.

Felix Hoffmann retired in 1928 and spent his final days in Switzerland, dabbling in art history. He never became a household name for his contribution to the world's medicine cabinets, but the dye-and-pharmaceutical company he worked for certainly did: Farbenfabriken vorm. Friedr. Bayer & Co., now known as Bayer.

ASPIRIN'S COMING-OF-AGE IN AMERICA

When Aspirin found its way to America at the beginning of the twentieth century, the nation's citizens were in dire need of better health. A person born in 1900 could only expect to live to be forty-seven years old.

The top three causes of death were infections: pneumonia, tuberculosis, and enteritis, a diarrhea-triggering infection of the digestive tract typically caused by contaminated food or water. These diseases killed nearly one in three Americans.

Today's leading killers—heart disease and cancer—were less-common causes of death (at fourth and seventh place, respectively).

The available medical treatments at the time, you may not be surprised to learn, leaned toward the ineffective. In 1980, a researcher combed through a common 1927 medical textbook and found that a mere *6 percent* of treatments it recommended were considered to be effective by more modern standards.

The first edition of the *Merck Manual*—which is still produced as a popular reference book that provides an overview of standard treatments for a variety of conditions—reveals that many medicines and remedies in 1899 range from humorous to downright scary.

For example, acceptable treatments for headache included arsenic; a plaster of capsicum (hot pepper) on the nape of the neck; coffee and morphine; electric shocks; and for those severe headaches, leeches behind the ears.

Common arthritis treatments also included arsenic, as well as numerous types of mercury, which is now known to be highly toxic in most of its forms.

Little wonder that one Harvard doctor remarked that it was only "somewhere between 1910 and 1912 (that) a random patient with a random disease, consulting a doctor chosen at random, had, for the first time in the history of mankind, a better than fifty-fifty chance of profiting from the encounter."

It's also not surprising that aspirin found an audience of patients and physicians around the world eager to embrace more effective medications.

"Drug companies at the time were trying to produce purified, standardized medications. It was an era, at the turn of the century, when pharmacology was becoming more of a science, and where physicians were starting to look at the old drugs that they had been using to see if they were still worth using, and also at what new drugs might be available," says Jan McTavish, Ph.D., an assistant professor of history in the department of social sciences at Alcorn State University in Mississippi, and author of *Pain and Profits* (Rutgers University Press, 2004), a history of headache remedies.

"The previous forms of therapy were based on the concept of balance: You have too much of something in your body, so you take a drug that will rid you of that substance. Almost all drugs were some form of 'puke or purge,' quite literally," she says. "The toxicity of some of those things was noted, but in the absence of something to substitute, they kept using them because they didn't want to *not* use them."

Bayer blazed new trails with its drug in the way it patented its process and promoted Aspirin, Dr. McTavish says. Previously, only snake-oil salesmen patented their dubious "medicines." Real, legitimate drug makers just didn't do this. Nor did they advertise directly to consumers, which Bayer would eventually do.

Though the drug immediately enjoyed uninterrupted success, developments wouldn't remain so kind to its parent company.

During World War I, British authorities feared they'd lose access to supplies of the drug, so they launched a search for a non-German source of Aspirin, offering a handsome cash reward to whoever could develop a way to manufacture it. An Australian pharmacist won the contest and named his drug Aspro.

Also during the war, the U.S. government seized the company's American assets. In late 1918, it auctioned off Bayer's American properties. A small West Virginia firm that peddled patent medicines for dandruff and impotence, Sterling Products, bought the assets for $5.3 million. For more than seventy years to follow, each company would be making Bayer aspirin.

A few years later the U.S. authorities decided that the name "Aspirin" had become so commonly used that it was part of the public domain. Thus, in the United States—as well as in the United Kingdom and France—aspirin is a generic drug name, with a lowercase spelling, which refers to acetylsalicylic acid, and a number of companies make it. But in more than seventy countries around the world, the Bayer company still has the trademark rights to the name, and is the sole maker of Aspirin.

By the 1920s, scientific studies had firmly established the usefulness of aspirin for bringing down high fevers. By the 1950s, it was scientifically proven to be an effective and safe pain reliever for headache, arthritis, muscle pain, menstrual pain, and dental pain.

As the 1900s progressed, landmark improvements in public health and medicine added years, then decades, to the average American's life expectancy. These included the widespread use of vaccines against smallpox, diphtheria, polio, and other infectious diseases that killed tens of thousands each year. Chlorinated drinking water, better sewage-disposal methods, food-safety improvements, and public education campaigns to improve the public's hygiene reduced the spread of disease even further.

Another development that changed the face of health in America, which was nothing short of monumental, was the discovery of penicillin. This drug was accidentally born in 1928 in an English laboratory when bacteriologist Alexander Fleming noticed that *Penicillium* mold contamination had destroyed an area of bacterial growth in a culture dish left in a lab sink. By 1945, penicillin was widely available to the public.

The discovery has been called possibly "the moment when the practice of medicine left the Dark Ages." The drug marked the first time that mankind could once and for all defeat microscopic bugs that caused so much human suffering and death.

But as all these developments added to people's life expectancy, the burden of diseases associated with older age became more prominent. Heart disease became the leading cause of death in the United States in 1921, and strokes rose to the third-leading cause of death in 1938—and both have retained these positions ever since.

Today heart disease claims roughly 700,000 lives in America each year, and strokes kill another 160,000. And the number of people who are *living* with these conditions is truly staggering: Thirteen million Americans have coronary heart disease, in which they have poor blood flow to their hearts, and nearly seven million have angina, the chest pain caused by that lack of blood flow. Plus, nearly 700,000 Americans each year have a stroke.

Another disease with a heavy toll in modern life is cancer. Roughly 1.3 million Americans developed cancer in 2004, a figure that excludes more than a million cases of skin cancer, and roughly 560,000 died from various cancers that year.

Yet another condition striking in epidemic numbers is diabetes. A condition associated in many cases with obesity and lack of physical activity, diabetes affects more than eighteen million Americans. The disease makes a person more likely to have heart disease or stroke and develop eye, foot, nerve, and kidney damage.

Adding to the list of today's worrisome health concerns is Alzheimer's disease, a disorienting, disabling condition of the aged, which is a serious cause for concern as an unprecedented wave of Baby Boomers head into their elder years.

But guess what? Aspirin, still the most widely used pain reliever in the world, has stepped up to the plate and is demonstrating its usefulness as a proven—or possible—treatment and preventive approach for all of these conditions . . . and more.

ASPIRIN'S SECOND CENTURY

For a drug that's chugging into its second one hundred years of use, aspirin looks remarkably attractive to scientists seeking answers to today's threats. Researchers have published more than 27,000 scientific articles that study the drug (*way* more, in fact, since that number was from 1997).

"It was the wonder drug of the twentieth century and it's likely to be the wonder drug of the twenty-first century," says Charles Hennekens, M.D., Dr.P.H., an epidemiologist (someone who studies patterns of human disease) and former Harvard researcher who held a leadership role in a landmark study begun in the 1980s that was the first to reveal aspirin as a powerful tool in preventing a first heart attack.

Almost 50,000 tons of acetylsalicylic acid are made each year; Americans pop roughly 80 million aspirin tablets *each day*.

A major part of its appeal is its price. Inexpensive and easily available, aspirin offers a simple way to head off diseases that become extremely expensive and difficult to treat once they've fully erupted and require high-tech tests and treatments. That's a significant plus nowadays when the American health system is in crisis and so many people are uninsured and can't afford medical treatment.

The drug's cardiovascular benefits and easy affordability will also make it more important in many poorer countries around the world in coming years, as their residents find themselves embarking on the longevity trend that America enjoyed in the 1900s, Dr. Hennekens says. Namely, countries like China are increasing their life expectancy by conquering malnutrition and infections. This means more and more people will be living longer, but developing heart disease, stroke, and cancer in rising numbers, especially as their citizens are adopting an unhealthy Western lifestyle by doing things like taking up smoking, eating a high-fat diet, and doing less physical activity.

The fact that scientists are finding, so deep into aspirin's life span, that it can help prevent these diseases makes it an unusual find.

"It's kind of weird to have a drug this many years later where we still learn so many things about it," says Steven Weisman, Ph.D., head of global health-care products at Innovative Science Solutions in Morristown, New Jersey. A pharmaceutical consultant, Dr. Weisman has worked as an executive for several aspirin companies, including Bayer.

"It's a drug that has had nine lives. When the thing was introduced, people died in their forties and so they didn't have the emergence of heart disease yet, so there was no way to even think about that potential benefit. Now we're at a different time and place, and it's neat that aspirin kind of matured along with us and it's still able to provide important benefits," he says.

He foresees even more decades of discoveries into the drug's actions and abilities. Aspirin's main activity in the body was only discovered in the 1970s (we'll get into that in more detail in the next chapter) but it may work in other ways that are still a mystery.

"We'll probably go into the next decade much more worried about immune-related diseases and diseases of heredity like Alzheimer's, and it certainly looks like aspirin may have a place in those as well," Dr. Weisman predicts.

This book will delve into the developing uses for aspirin, which include these life-threatening conditions and others that may surprise you, including fertility and pregnancy issues. We'll also discuss its everyday uses, such as relieving headaches and fever, so you can make sure you're using your aspirin to its greatest effectiveness.

If you've skimmed this far into the book but feel you can't reap the benefits of this drug since you count among the percentage of people who can't take aspirin due to its side effects, read on.

Doctors are finding new ways to make aspirin available even to people who have digestive bleeding or asthma problems triggered by the drug. And new formulations of aspirin are under investigation to reduce the stomach irritation it causes.

But before we talk about all the many ways that aspirin can improve your health, let's take a look at how this miracle drug works its wonders in your body.

2

How It Works

 Shake a generic, inexpensive tablet of aspirin into your hand, and you'll have good reason to wonder what all the fuss is about.

The round shape and plain white surface you're likely examining don't give the appearance of a versatile medication. You can buy it in the grocery store near the mouthwash and foot powder . . . not a particularly honored home for a wonder drug of the ages. And the greatest mystery it would seem to hold is how to get past the child-safety mechanism on some bottles.

Looks can be deceiving. In reality, when you swallow a tablet of this familiar drug, it slips into a fascinating dance that whirls and swirls throughout your bloodstream, affecting tissues and organs all around your body. But for generations, no one really knew how aspirin worked.

Scientists and consumers knew it was effective in easing pain and lowering fever, but they had no idea how.

Then in the early 1970s, aspirin started proving to be more exciting. The late British pharmacologist John Vane and colleagues discovered how the drug exerts its effects in the body. (Actually, they were experimenting with guinea-pig lungs, but the information proved to be applicable to humans.) The finding was important enough to earn Vane a Nobel Prize in 1982. Sorry, that's *Sir* Vane—he was also knighted for his contributions to medicine. He died in late 2004.

The discovery opened the door to a greater understanding of how the body's internal processes contribute to heart disease and other serious diseases. It also paved the way for a group of newer, much more expensive drugs that captured headlines in the late 1990s for their ability to treat arthritis and other painful conditions without as many side effects as aspirin causes in some people.

To understand how aspirin could help add decades to your life— and more enjoyment to your later years—it's helpful to know how it works. Other than involving a few long words, the tale of what aspirin does in your body is actually pretty simple.

In fact, it can be told in just a few paragraphs.

How Aspirin Works: The Short Story

You have very busy substances called *prostaglandins* that work all around your body. These are made in most or all of the types of cells in your body and act upon the cells that made them and surrounding cells. They play all kinds of roles—some that contribute to good health, some that don't, and some that can go either way depending on the situation.

"Prostaglandins are really important in many different body functions, from helping us raise our temperature if we have an infection, to causing pain so we avoid things that are dangerous to us, regulating the menstrual cycle, regulating kidney function, and regulating stomach integrity," says Steven Weisman, Ph.D., an aspirin researcher, pharmacologist, and consultant with Innovative Science Solutions in New Jersey.

> **In case the word prostaglandins makes you think of the prostate gland, you're on to something; they were first isolated from semen (they make the muscle contract in the uterus), and experts thought they originated in the gland.**

Prostaglandins are also involved in your body's natural inflammatory response that helps heal injuries, and they help your blood clot.

Aspirin, however, reduces the amount of prostaglandins in your system, therefore reducing pain and inflammation and helping your blood flow freely. It's that simple. "Almost all the good things from aspirin, as well as bad things from aspirin, are related to a single mechanism," Dr. Weisman says.

If that's as deeply as you care to delve into how aspirin works, that's fine. You can enjoy the rest of the book based on this knowledge.

But if you examine aspirin's effects a little more thoroughly, the extra details you'll find are pretty cool, too. Knowing more about how aspirin works will help you better understand later in the book how it might help protect you from heart disease, cancer, Alzheimer's, and other conditions.

HOW ASPIRIN WORKS: THE LONGER STORY

The Aspirin Vocabulary

- *Arachidonic acid.* This is a fatty acid, and a variety of events will trigger your body's cells to release it from their membranes, allowing it to be converted into prostaglandins.
- *Cyclooxygenase.* This enzyme, better known as COX, plays a key role in converting arachidonic acid into prostaglandins. Aspirin takes COX out of commission, lessening prostaglandin production. COX comes in two forms that we'll focus on in this book: COX-1, which is found constantly around your body and is involved in processes that keep your system working properly; and COX-2, which is generally scarce during normal conditions, but crops up in greater amounts during particular events, such as during inflammation.

- *Prostaglandins.* Hormones produced by most, if not all, cells in your body. These have a number of effects in your body, some that are a benefit to your health by protecting normal bodily function, and some that can be harmful.
- *Thromboxane A2.* Made from a prostaglandin, this substance is produced by platelets in your blood, prompting them to clump together and form blood clots.

When you toss back an aspirin tablet, it doesn't waste any time getting to work. In one study, researchers could find aspirin in the fluid in people's joints just ten to thirty minutes after they took the drug.

Your body absorbs between 80 to 100 percent of the drug from your digestive system, and it quickly spreads throughout most of the tissues and fluids in your body. It reaches its peak levels in your body within an hour or two after you take it. However, this varies on the type of aspirin you take. If the aspirin has an enteric coating, which lets it slip past your stomach before it breaks down, you absorb it more slowly. If you drink a fizzy aspirin dissolved in water, you absorb it more quickly.

It moves out of your body quickly, too. Half the dose is eliminated in your urine within two to four hours if you take a low dose, or fifteen to thirty hours if you take a high dose. If you're breast-feeding, salicylate from the aspirin also comes out in your breast milk.

Once it spreads throughout your body, it creates its beneficial effects—as well as its unwanted side effects—by interfering with one of your body's natural processes.

The COX Factor

The raw material that is used to make prostaglandins is an essential fatty acid called *arachidonic acid.* The process that turns arachidonic acid into prostaglandins is the crucial step where aspirin works its wonders.

An enzyme called cyclooxygenase (pronounced sy-klow-oxygenase), or COX, is needed to turn the arachidonic acid found in cells' surfaces into prostaglandins. When COX is disabled, it can't make prostaglandins.

That's what aspirin does—it prevents the COX enzyme from helping generate prostaglandins. In chapter 1, you learned that Felix Hoffmann, who discovered a way to produce aspirin in 1897, made it by *acetylating*—or adding an acetyl molecule—to a chemical called salicylic acid, which is naturally found in willows and other plants. Thus, the resulting aspirin is chemically known as acetylsalicylic acid.

Hoffmann originally came up with this formulation to make the drug easier on the stomach and be better absorbed so it would have more medicinal effect. However, this is also what makes aspirin work so well. When it gets into your system, the aspirin is split up and the acetyl molecule gets tacked onto COX enzymes, permanently preventing them from producing prostaglandins.

Aspirin belongs to a family of drugs called nonsteroidal antiinflammatory drugs (NSAIDs); the other over-the-counter NSAIDs are ibuprofen (such as Advil), ketoprofen (Orudis), and naproxen (Aleve). Aspirin is the only one of these that permanently takes COX out of action. The others inhibit it, but the effect is reversible.

Even though the salicylic acid in certain plants fascinated healers and chemists for centuries, that component of the aspirin now isn't considered to be particularly helpful. Salicylic acid can dampen inflammation, but weakly, and its effect on the COX enzyme rapidly wears off, says Garret FitzGerald, M.D., a professor of pharmacology and cardiovascular medicine at the University of Pennsylvania, who studies how drugs inhibit COX. Instead, it's the acetyl portion of the drug that's mostly to thank for aspirin's effectiveness.

The Benefits of Blocking COX

Reducing prostaglandin production is how aspirin decreases inflammation, since this process depends on these chemicals. Less inflammation means less pain. Aspirin's anti-inflammatory action may also be how it can reduce the risk of cancer and Alzheimer's disease, since inflammation can play a role in these diseases.

Aspirin also reduces pain by interfering with prostaglandin production, since prostaglandins make pain receptors in your body more sensitive and easily bothered. Simply applying prostaglandins to a person's skin can cause a painful sensation.

And aspirin reduces fever through the same mechanism. A prostaglandin dials up the internal "thermostat" in your brain to a higher temperature when you have an infection. Aspirin keeps this from happening. It also helps reduce your temperature by causing blood vessels to dilate, allowing more blood to flow out to the periphery of your body, helping you dissipate heat.

Yet another way aspirin helps your body is by reducing your blood's ability to clot. This is one of the drug's *major* health-protecting powers. As you'll see in the next sections, blood clots create havoc in your body—sometimes fatal—by taking unwanted trips through blood vessels and contributing to heart attacks and strokes.

Circulating in your blood are tiny structures called platelets. They're actually broken-down fragments of a larger type of blood cell, and the platelets survive for about ten days. Platelets help your blood form clots by clumping together.

Each platelet contains the COX enzyme, which the platelets use to produce a substance called *thromboxane A2,* which is made from a prostaglandin. It helps platelets stick together. Once they stick together, they start producing other chemicals that have kind of a snowballing effect in encouraging even more blood clotting. But aspirin keeps the platelets from forming thromboxane, nipping this process in the bud.

Aspirin permanently puts the kibosh on the COX enzyme in the platelets, mostly as the drug is in your gut and it's exposed to platelets whisking through the blood vessels in the area.

And once a platelet loses its ability to clot, it's permanently grounded from joining up with its friends; for the rest of a roughly ten-day life span, it will not be taking part in any clots. You'll bleed more readily for up to eight days or so after you take an aspirin as your body gradually replaces old platelets that were affected by the aspirin. That's why you need to stop taking aspirin a week or so before surgery, to cut down on excessive bleeding, unless your doctor directs you otherwise.

Unfortunately, COX isn't always the bad guy that needs to be knocked out. In some instances, it actually plays a role in *protecting* your body. That's where the less pleasant effects of aspirin can come into play.

Aspirin's Actions Get Complicated

Your stomach produces hydrochloric acid and enzymes, which break down your food and destroy wayward bacteria that have gotten into your digestive system.

This harsh liquid is strong enough to burn into bodily tissue. So what keeps your stomach from digesting itself? Normally the contents can't harm the sensitive lining of your stomach because cells in your stomach generate mucus, which forms a gel-like barrier against the acid.

Prostaglandins are involved in protecting the stomach by a number of possible means, including inhibiting acid production, increasing blood flow, increasing mucus production, upping the secretion of protective bicarbonate, and speeding up the turnover of cells in the stomach lining.

When you take an aspirin and it disables the COX in the lining of your stomach, the resulting drop in prostaglandins leaves your stomach less protected. Hence, you can develop ulcers in the stomach lining and bleeding in your digestive tract. Even if you take aspirin into your body via a suppository (yes, it's available in that form), it can still cause stomach damage through this process, even though it never goes through your stomach.

Taking an aspirin by mouth can also directly cause temporary damage to your stomach; when the pill touches the surface of the organ, it can leave a little eroded spot, which might bleed briefly.

Aspirin tablets that are *enteric-coated* are covered with a special layer that allows them to pass through your stomach unchanged, and they dissolve when they reach your small intestine. This keeps the aspirin from causing the direct irritation in your stomach, but once it dissolves into your system, it can still cause the reduction in prostaglandins that protect your stomach, resulting in damage.

Pharmaceutical companies unveiled several new anti-inflammatory medications in the late 1990s in an attempt to come up with a drug that targets the "bad" prostaglandins and spares the "good" ones. These include rofecoxib (Vioxx) and celecoxib (Celebrex).

The Many Faces of COX

The substance that helps produce prostaglandins, the COX enzyme, actually comes in several forms, COX-1 and COX-2, which have different jobs in the body. (A third form is being investigated, but we'll just focus on the first two here.)

COX-1 is always present in a "housekeeping" role, ensuring that your body's processes work consistently and properly. It's the version involved in protecting the stomach and making your blood clot. COX-2, however, is normally present in a limited amount only in certain places in your body, but bursts onto the scene on special occasions, such as during inflammation. Aspirin affects both types of COX—COX-1 more than COX-2, making it a "nonspecific inhibitor." This is good since it keeps blood from clotting and dampens inflammation; not so good in that it impairs your stomach's protective processes.

The newer anti-inflammatory drugs, such as rofecoxib (Vioxx) and celecoxib (Celebrex), which are used to treat osteoarthritis and other painful conditions, are known as COX-2 inhibitors. These target COX-2—thus preventing the harmful prostaglandins that it helps produce—while sparing COX-1. In theory, this should allow the drug to cause fewer side effects in the digestive system.

These drugs, though, can have their shortcomings. In September 2004, the pharmaceutical company Merck & Co. stopped selling Vioxx. A long-term study investigating the drug's ability to prevent the recurrence of colon polyps (you'll see why this seems like a good idea later in the book) found that people taking the drug for more than eighteen months had an unacceptably higher risk of heart attacks and strokes, though their risk was still small. This wasn't the first time that research had found a higher risk of cardiovascular disease in people taking the drug. The incident raised a call for drug experts to look into the possible harmful effects on the heart of other COX-2 inhibitors, too.

Even if Vioxx comes back on the market and its COX-2 inhibiting relatives remain available, the study's black eye isn't the only thing going against them.

They're also expensive—a bottle containing thirty Celebrex pills can cost $80, based on a price listing at a popular Internet-based pharmacy. You can buy a bottle of one thousand store-brand aspirin at the pharmacy or supermarket for less than $10.

Also, though these drugs can reduce pain and inflammation, they don't keep your blood from clotting, since that's a function of the COX-1 enzyme, which these drugs don't target. Therefore, they don't offer protection against cardiovascular disease like aspirin does. Finally, they're not completely without the gastrointestinal side effects that aspirin can cause. They, too, can cause gastrointestinal damage and bleeding.

Also, many experts feel that aspirin has special abilities through processes that don't involve prostaglandins, but will require more research to uncover.

For more information on COX-2 inhibitors, see the heart disease and cancer chapters. To learn more about how to safely take aspirin with less stomach irritation and other irritation, be sure to read chapter 13.

Section II

Protecting Your Cardiovascular System

In this section, you'll learn how aspirin affects your cardiovascular system, which is your heart and the blood vessels connected to it. Your heart acts like a pump, sending vital blood out through these tube-like vessels to all parts of your body.

Your blood, of course, is normally a fluid, and it flows easily through this system. However, sometimes it forms clots, which can interfere with the smooth flow of blood. If you've ever had a stopped-up water pipe in your house, you know that the results can range from aggravating to catastrophic.

The same happens if one of your body's "pipes" becomes clogged. The results can be dangerous or fatal.

Thankfully, aspirin is an inexpensive, reliable way to help keep your blood flowing and your cardiovascular system working properly.

3

Heart Health

Aspirin makers were long concerned that the medication might somehow be harmful to the heart.

After it was discovered (technically, *re*discovered) in Bayer's laboratories, the promising new drug lingered in limbo for more than a year in the late 1890s because the company's director of pharmacological research feared that it could weaken customers' hearts. He may have had this erroneous belief because, at the time, people who used salicylic acid—a forerunner of aspirin—commonly took it in huge doses that made them short of breath and caused their hearts to beat rapidly.

Another Bayer scientist, however, tried it on himself, then snuck the drug out to German doctors on the sly to offer to their patients. When it turned out not to be toxic to anyone's heart, the company decided to develop it.

Even a half-century later, aspirin makers were still taking pains to assure the public about aspirin's heart safety, says epidemiologist and longtime aspirin researcher Charles Hennekens, M.D., Dr.P.H., a former Harvard professor, aspirin expert, and current visiting professor at the University of Miami School of Medicine and Florida Atlantic University.

He keeps an aspirin advertisement that ran in the *Journal of the American Medical Association* in the 1950s, which featured a block of text set aside in a box that reassured that it doesn't affect the heart.

But in the late 1940s, doctors started encountering signs that aspirin indeed can affect the heart—but not in the way that manufacturers had feared.

A California ear, nose, and throat doctor named Lawrence Craven noticed a curious fact about some of his tonsillectomy patients. When he gave patients gum containing aspirin for pain relief, those who chewed large amounts of the medication tended to bleed excessively.

Acting on a hunch, in 1948 he started treating his older male patients with aspirin to prevent heart attacks. In the mid-1950s, he published several papers announcing that none of the 8,000-plus patients on aspirin had suffered a heart attack, and that the aspirin had completely protected them from strokes, too.

He was ahead of his time. Unfortunately for the legacy of Dr. Craven, his study data were crude and he published his findings in medical journals that weren't widely read, thus people paid little attention to his findings. Neither did it help his cause when he died of a heart attack in 1957.

ASPIRIN ENTERS THE HEART-PROTECTING ERA

In 1971, scientists learned that aspirin works to keep platelets in the blood from clotting, an action that could be construed as protective of the heart. However, during that decade, randomized trials investigating whether aspirin could reduce the risk of second heart attacks came up with conflicting results, probably because the trials were too small in size.

These early trials chose to look at people who'd *already* had heart attacks or strokes since they'd be more likely to have another heart attack in the near future, which then would more quickly show the researchers whether the aspirin was helping.

By 1985, the evidence was strong enough that the FDA approved the use of aspirin for preventing heart attacks in people who had already had one or who had a condition called "unstable angina." Angina is chest pain caused by insufficient blood flow to the heart, and unstable angina is more frequent and severe than regular angina.

In 1988, the benefit of aspirin in preventing a first heart attack was demonstrated conclusively in the Physicians' Health Study. This was a major research project led by Dr. Hennekens that involved more than 22,000 apparently healthy male doctors as subjects. It investigated whether aspirin would help prevent cardiovascular disease and also looked into whether the nutrient beta-carotene would help prevent cancer.

The Aspirin Vocabulary

- *Angina.* Discomfort in your chest that results from a lack of sufficient blood flow to your heart muscle.
- *Atherosclerosis.* The condition marked by plaque buildup in artery walls. It makes the artery harder and narrower and interferes with proper blood flow through the vessel.
- *Cardiovascular.* Refers to your heart, arteries, veins, and other blood vessels.
- *Coronary arteries.* The vessels that supply oxygen-laden blood to your heart muscle.
- *Coronary heart disease.* The condition in which your heart isn't getting enough oxygen-bearing blood because the coronary arteries are narrowed with plaque. This can lead to a heart attack. Also known as coronary artery disease.
- *Heart attack.* An event that causes permanent damage to an area of your heart muscle due to lack of sufficient oxygen to the area. This usually involves a blood clot forming in an artery that feeds blood to the heart, which is already narrow due to growth of plaque in the artery. A heart attack is sometimes called a myocardial infarction.
- *Plaque.* An accumulation of fat, cholesterol, and other substances in the wall of an artery. Also known as an *atheroma.*

Coordinated by the Harvard Medical School and Brigham and Women's Hospital in Boston, the project was a *randomized double-blind placebo-controlled trial*. This means that some subjects received aspirin, beta-carotene, or both, and some received placebos—a neutral substance with no medicinal value. The double-blind aspect means that neither the investigators nor the subjects knew who was getting which, to minimize the chance of reporting benefits or risks based on knowledge of the treatment.

After five years of treatment and follow-up, the project hit a surprising interruption in 1988. The safety board overseeing the project ordered the aspirin portion to be halted, since it wouldn't be ethical to continue: There was a 44 percent reduction in risk of a first heart attack among the aspirin takers. The benefit was so great that the researchers could no longer withhold aspirin from people who weren't receiving it.

Nowadays, it's an accepted fact that "For secondary prevention (preventing follow-up heart attacks) there's no question. The evidence is

Diabetes Creates a Special Need for Aspirin

Nearly two-thirds of people with diabetes die of heart disease or stroke. Middle-aged people with diabetes are two to four times as likely to have coronary artery disease, stroke, or peripheral arterial disease as people without diabetes—and an equally higher risk of dying in general.

Atherosclerosis, or plaque accumulation in arteries, and blood clotting are major contributors to the risk of these conditions. Lab tests have found that platelets in people with diabetes clot more easily, and researchers have found extra-high levels of thromboxane in people with type 2 diabetes and cardiovascular disease. This is a substance related to prostaglandin that causes platelets to clump together.

Thus, according to the American Diabetes Association, diabetics have an increased need to add aspirin to their daily health-maintenance regimens. In 2004, the organization issued a position statement recommending 75 to 162 milligrams of aspirin daily in diabetic men and women with a history of heart attack, bypass procedures, stroke or transient ischemic attack, peripheral arterial disease, claudication (leg pain), or angina, in order to prevent secondary cardiovascular events. This is, of course, only for those who don't have a bleeding problem, aspirin allergy, recent gastrointestinal bleeding, active liver disease, or who are taking anticoagulants (blood thinners).

The organization also recommends this daily dosage to prevent *first* cardiovascular events in people with type 2 diabetes if they're over forty or have added risk factors, such as high blood pressure, smoking, unhealthy cholesterol, or a family history of cardiovascular disease. These recommendations don't extend to young people under the age of twenty-one, due to concerns about Reye's syndrome (see page 168).

clear and very overwhelming" in support of aspirin's usefulness, says Michael Lauer, M.D., the director of clinical research in the department of cardiovascular medicine at the Cleveland Clinic in Cleveland, Ohio.

The American Heart Association now recommends that most people who've had a heart attack or have unstable angina take aspirin to reduce their risk of future problems. We'll talk more about how you should use aspirin to prevent a secondary heart attack later in this chapter.

Before that, we'll discuss the newer research supporting the Physicians' Health Study, which shows that you don't have to wait to have a heart attack before you can start making use of aspirin's protective effects: Even if you feel fine now, taking aspirin might make you less likely to have a *first* heart attack.

But first let's talk about how the heart works, what sorts of problems make it go astray, and how aspirin can help keep it pumping properly.

How Your Heart Works (or Doesn't Work)

Your heart, which weighs about nine ounces, is a hollow, muscular organ containing four chambers. The heart's job is to pump your blood to your lungs—where it picks up oxygen from the air you breathe—then

Aspirin Offers Another Tool for Heart Surgeons

Even cutting-edge, high-tech procedures to treat heart disease can use a helping hand from good old aspirin.

One way to open up clogged coronary arteries is to do an angioplasty. This involves running a thin tube through an artery in the groin or arm to the clogged coronary artery. When the catheter is in place, the doctor inflates a balloon at the end. This pushes aside the plaque blocking the artery, allowing blood to flow through.

Often the procedure also involves a stent, or spring-like sleeve, which is placed around the balloon. As the balloon inflates, it expands the stent to hold back the plaque after the catheter is removed, reducing the chances of the artery narrowing down at that spot again.

The American College of Cardiology (ACC) and the American Heart Association (AHA) recommend a dose of 80 to 325 milligrams of aspirin at least two hours before the procedure to reduce the risk of blood clots after the procedure. Another antiplatelet drug called clopidogrel (Plavix) is also a standard drug used before the procedure, and for daily use for a few weeks after stent placement.

Aspirin also can play an important role in a surgery called "coronary artery bypass grafting," or CABG (pronounced cabbage) for short. During this procedure, which President Bill Clinton underwent in 2004, doctors attach another blood vessel to a blocked coronary artery so that the blood "bypasses" the blockage through the new vessel. Earlier in the procedure's history, doctors removed an expendable vein from the leg—the saphenous vein—to use for the bypass. This vein is still used in CABGs, but doctors now also use an artery from inside the chest wall.

In 2004, the ACC and the AHA issued joint guidelines urging the use of aspirin after CABG surgery. A daily dose of 100 to 325 milligrams, started soon after the surgery, helps keep the grafted vessel open after the procedure and can reduce the risk of death, heart attack, stroke, and kidney failure after the surgery. It should be continued "indefinitely," the organizations advise.

on through your arteries to the furthest reaches of your body so it can pass the vital oxygen it contains to your cells and pick up their wastes. Your heart then pumps the blood back through your veins so it can again pick up oxygen from your lungs.

Each day, your heart pumps the equivalent of 2,000 gallons of blood through your body's 60,000 *miles* of blood vessels. It's a repetitive job, but a healthy heart has no problem with the routine.

For all the important work it does, your heart is sort of short-changed. Every cell in your body needs oxygen to function. The cells in your heart are no exception. But all that blood that passes through it doesn't directly provide the heart muscle with oxygen! The lining of the heart won't let blood seep into the thick muscular walls of the organ. Thus, the heart depends on its *coronary arteries* for a supply of oxygen to keep the muscle healthy.

When oxygen-laden blood heads out to the body from the heart, it exits the heart through the aorta. Some of this blood immediately flows into the coronary arteries, which branch off the aorta just outside the heart. The coronary arteries cling to the surface of the heart, and tinier vessels branch off them and head into the walls of the organ.

Coronary heart disease arises when the normal flow of blood through the coronary arteries is slowed or interrupted. The underlying problem contributing to this is the buildup of a fatty substance called *plaque* inside the artery walls. This process of buildup is called atherosclerosis, which comes from the Greek terms for "paste" and "hardness."

We will now turn the discussion over to David F. Kong, M.D., a Duke University cardiologist and assistant professor, who has studied aspirin and has a colorful manner of describing heart disease.

The fatty plaques have cholesterol in them, they have flecks of calcium in them, they have some cellular debris in them, and they have little oily lakes inside them. Sometimes the plaque is stringy, or flaky, or puffy, or squishy. And the stuff basically is covered with a thin sheet of cells.

As long as these cells are intact, then the elements of blood that respond to injury say "Okay, it's a happy day." But when plaque *ruptures*—when it becomes unstable and the thin layer of cells that covers it is disrupted—all of a sudden it starts an alarm. It's like when you cut yourself, you disrupt the cells in the blood vessels in your skin. The blood says "Aha, there's an injury happening, we need to form a clot." When the plaque ruptures, then the elements in the blood that are responsible for blood-clot formation also say "We need to form a clot."

When plaque simply builds up in your arteries and slows the flow of blood to your heart, it's known as *coronary artery disease* or *coronary heart disease.* The decreased blood flow to your heart can cause an uncomfortable pressure or squeezing sensation in your chest, but you may also feel pain in your neck or jaw, shoulder, back, or arm. This is called *angina.* It may only occur during periods of activity or stress, but the more serious unstable form flares up when you're at rest.

When a plaque ruptures and a clot forms on it, blocking the flow of blood through the already-narrow artery, then you're having a heart attack. You may also see this referred to as a *myocardial infarction;* the heart muscle is your myocardium, and the permanent tissue damage in the muscle resulting from lack of blood is called an infarction or infarct.

That clot—more precisely *avoiding* that clot—is one way that aspirin comes into the picture. As you learned in chapter 2, aspirin permanently prevents elements in your blood called platelets from being able to latch onto one another and form a clot. A platelet lives for ten days or so, and once the aspirin shuts off its clotting ability, it doesn't regain it. The aspirin helps your blood flow more smoothly past any plaque that's narrowing an artery, and should a plaque rupture, the aspirin will reduce the chance of a clot clinging to it. These actions help ensure that your heart receives the constant nourishing supply of oxygen it requires.

Aspirin may also help prevent heart disease by its anti-inflammatory ability. The process in which plaque accumulates in your arteries isn't just a simple plumbing issue, like gunk building up in the pipes under your kitchen sink. Inflammation also plays a role.

Inflammation is involved throughout the process of plaque accumulation. It begins when something inflames the inner lining of an artery. The culprit behind the inflammation could be LDL cholesterol—the

When You're Having a Heart Attack

If you think you're having a heart attack, your first step should be to reach for a phone and call 911. Then be ready to take aspirin.

The American Heart Association made an official statement in 1997 advocating the use of aspirin in "virtually all patients" to treat an evolving acute myocardial infarction (in other words, a heart attack as it's happening).

An important study of 17,000 men and women found that those who took 162 milligrams of aspirin within twenty-four hours of a heart attack and continued for a month were 23 percent less likely to die of heart-related disease than people who'd taken a placebo.

According to the Mayo Clinic, if you think you're having a heart attack, you should first call 911 or, if you don't have 911 service in your area, call the emergency response number that is available. Don't try to drive yourself to the hospital or have a friend or family member drive you—emergency medical responders are equipped to take care of you on the way to the hospital.

Then take 162 milligrams of aspirin. Chew the tablet or tablets first so you absorb them more quickly. The aspirin will help reduce clotting in your blood and enable it to get past obstacles in the arteries feeding your heart. Be sure to let the first responders know that you've taken the medication.

Warning signs of heart attack include:

- An uncomfortable squeezing or pressure in the center of your chest. It may be a steady or intermittent sensation.
- Pain or discomfort in one or both arms, as well as your stomach, back, neck, or jaw.
- Shortness of breath, sweating, light-headedness, or dizziness.

"bad" kind—that has been altered by free radicals, the rogue oxygen molecules that zip through your system creating havoc. Or the source of the problem could be a bacteria or virus.

In response to the inflammation, white blood cells, which are part of your immune system, penetrate into the inner lining of the artery.

It's the COX-2s' Bad-News Blues

The drugs known as COX-2 inhibitors held great promise for pain sufferers after they hit the market in the late 1990s. Dubbed "super aspirin" by
some, they tackled pain and inflammation through an effect similar to aspirin's, but with less damage to the gastrointestinal tract.

However, in a startling move, Merck & Co. yanked its COX-2 inhibitor,
Vioxx, from the market in the fall of 2004, in the largest prescription-drug
withdrawal in history. Here's why:

While investigating the drug's use in people without known heart disease for preventing colon polyps, researchers noticed that too many
people were having heart attacks and strokes on the drug compared to
those taking a placebo; 3.5 percent versus 1.9 percent.

Many researchers had voiced concerns in the scientific literature
about this possible effect in previous years. In 2001, Eric Topol, M.D.,
chairman of the department of cardiovascular medicine of the Cleveland
Clinic, co-authored a paper claiming that Vioxx carried a five-times greater
heart attack risk than the over-the-counter NSAID naproxen, as he pointed
out in a blistering editorial in the *New York Times* on the heels of the recall.
He also took Merck and the FDA to task in an issue of the *New England
Journal of Medicine* that month over allowing the drug to hit the marketplace without properly investigating it.

The drug seems to have a harmful effect on the heart due to the way
it affects prostaglandins. Aspirin inhibits the production of a prostaglandin
relative called thromboxane and another chemical called prostacyclin.
Thromboxane is made by platelets and encourages clotting and blood-
vessel tightening, which is not helpful in terms of heart disease. Prostacyclin, made by cells lining blood vessels, has a counterbalancing effect,
inhibiting clotting and causing blood vessels to dilate.

Vioxx and the other COX-2 inhibitors inhibit prostacyclin but don't affect thromboxane, thus tipping the blood in favor of harmful clotting, wrote
Garret FitzGerald, M.D., of the University of Pennsylvania, Philadelphia,
in the same issue of the *New England Journal of Medicine*.

It remained to be seen whether other drugs in the family—Celebrex,

Bextra, and another that was under FDA consideration for approval—cause the same effects, but researchers needed to find out, both scientists wrote.

It's probably best for people with heart disease, or who are at high risk for it, to avoid these drugs for the time being. Michael Lauer, M.D., a colleague of Dr. Topol's, says he'd been advising patients in these groups for several years to avoid COX-2 inhibitors, particularly Vioxx.

This makes it easier for fats to accumulate in the vessel wall. This, in turn, sets the stage for snowballing accumulation of more immune cells, fat, and debris in the artery wall.

Later on, the growth of plaque that results from this process bulges out from the artery wall, obstructing blood flow. The growth is covered with a protective cap. However, inflammation can cause this cap to rupture, as Dr. Kong mentioned, exposing the contents to the bloodstream. A blood clot can form on this material, blocking the artery and triggering a heart attack.

Your doctor can do a simple blood test to check to see if you have inflammation going on in your body that could set the stage for heart disease. The test looks for a substance called C-reactive protein (CRP), which is produced by your liver when you have inflammation in your body. The American Heart Association and the Centers for Disease Control and Prevention recommend that you have the test done if your risk of developing heart disease in the next ten years is ten to 20 percent. You'll learn how to calculate your risk later in the chapter.

A study that followed more than 5,500 British men for twelve years found that the men in the group with the top one-third highest CRP levels were more than twice as likely to develop coronary heart disease as the men with the bottom third.

Another study looked at the relationship of aspirin to CRP and heart attack. It found that aspirin significantly reduced the risk of heart attack in the group of men with the highest CRP levels, but not in those with the lowest CRP levels.

ASPIRIN AND HEART DISEASE:
HELP FOR HEALTHY PEOPLE

In September 2003, the *Archives of Internal Medicine* published an analysis that pooled the results of the five published trials that had examined the effects of aspirin on primary heart-attack prevention. This type of study is called a *meta-analysis*.

These earlier trials, which included the Physicians' Health Study project that wrapped up early in 1988, included data from more than 55,000 apparently healthy men and women, says Dr. Hennekens, who was the lead researcher on the 2003 meta-analysis.

It found that aspirin use conclusively reduced the risk of having a first heart attack by about one third! The meta-analysis was unable to show significant links between aspirin and vascular-related *deaths* or stroke, probably because not enough of these events occurred in these studies to offer conclusive results.

The studies investigating aspirin use in healthy people have largely focused on men. That's due in part to the fact that middle-aged men are more likely to have heart attacks than middle-aged women, and researchers have studied the people who would have the most events to more quickly illustrate any abilities of aspirin, says Julie Buring, Sc.D., a professor of epidemiology at Harvard University, who is heading up a major project entitled the Women's Health Study. This project is looking at nearly 40,000 *female* health professionals to specifically investigate aspirin's ability to reduce the chances of first heart attacks and strokes in women.

Though the findings hadn't yet been published, Dr. Buring believes aspirin has the potential to help women lower their risk of a first heart attack or stroke, since the drug is well-established to be helpful for women in treating heart attacks while they're happening.

Despite such findings and recommendations from experts, surveys have noted that not enough people who could be benefiting from aspirin for their hearts are taking it. According to Dr. Hennekens, if more people who should be taking aspirin were actually doing so, it could prevent more than 10,000 premature deaths among patients with prior

Be Careful with Mixing and Matching Medications

One common over-the-counter pill, aspirin, can reduce your risk of a heart attack. But another, ibuprofen, may interfere with aspirin's protective effect if you take it regularly.

Aspirin helps prevent heart attacks by preventing platelets in the blood from clotting. As discussed in chapter 2, it does this by locking onto an enzyme in your body called cyclooxygenase, or COX. This disables the COX and prevents it from taking part in the production of a substance called thromboxane, which helps platelets stick together.

However, when you take ibuprofen first, it can occupy the little nook on the COX enzyme where the aspirin would have gone, and it keeps the aspirin from having its anticlotting effect.

However, just because this can be shown in blood samples in the laboratory doesn't necessarily mean that taking medications containing ibuprofen, such as Advil, will keep your aspirin from helping your heart, cautions Garret FitzGerald, M.D., a professor of pharmacology and cardiovascular medicine at the University of Pennsylvania.

Studies looking at groups of people to see if their aspirin and ibuprofen habits affect their chances of cardiovascular problems have found conflicting results. Some research links ibuprofen use to a greater chance of problems, and some doesn't.

Until larger studies provide more convincing answers on whether you can take ibuprofen if you're also taking aspirin for your heart, it's probably okay to take ibuprofen occasionally for pain, Dr. FitzGerald says. But if you need a pain-relieving drug regularly, you're probably better off taking one that shouldn't interfere, such as acetaminophen (Tylenol) or the prescription diclofenac (Cataflam).

heart attacks and strokes and more than 150,000 first heart attacks in the United States each year.

"We have underutilization of it in patient populations that would clearly benefit," Dr. Hennekens says. "If this drug were half as effective, ten times as expensive, and on prescription, maybe more people would take it more seriously," he joked. Aspirin is, after all, cheaply available in any supermarket near the shampoo and toothbrushes, rather than an exotic medication with a hard-to-pronounce name that you can only get from your physician. Maybe that makes it seem less valuable.

But another reason why some people are leery of tossing back aspirin for their hearts is that they fear the side effects. Since aspirin makes your blood flow more readily, it increases your risk of minor side effects like bruising and bleeding gums. More seriously, since aspirin also increases the risk that your stomach will become irritated by its own juices, it also creates the possibility that you'll develop gastrointestinal ulcers and bleeding.

These "bleeds" can be life-threatening, says Dr. Michael Lauer of the Cleveland Clinic. In fact, he's seen patients die of this type of bleeding. Another serious risk of aspirin is the chance it carries that you'll develop bleeding in the brain, which even in tiny amounts can cause "a devastating amount of damage," he says.

As a result, he says the take-home message is that "aspirin's not for everybody. We shouldn't be putting aspirin in the water supply like we use fluoride to prevent cavities."

You definitely don't want to take the risk of encountering these problems without good reason. However, Dr. Hennekens stresses the low chances of serious complications.

"Many people overestimate the side effects due to what they hear on TV or read in the newspapers. I think the side effects that are perceived by the public and doctors are much greater than the actual ones," he says.

In actuality, a 2004 meta-analysis in the *American Journal of Hematology* that looked at bleeding events associated with aspirin and many other drugs that reduce blood clotting found that low-dose aspirin—the sort recommended for preventing heart attacks—carried the lowest risk of all the drugs studied. In the roughly 12,600 patients who received this dose of aspirin in the studies, only 3.6 percent had bleeds of any kind, from minor to major.

Also, Dr. Hennekens points out, people involved in studies in which they *know* they're taking aspirin often report more side effects than in studies where they don't know if they're receiving the drug or the placebo. Most people know that aspirin can cause these sorts of side effects, and people may be more likely to notice bleeding problems when they're taking aspirin and associate them with the drug.

The whole decision of whether you should take aspirin to avoid a first heart attack, then, boils down to whether the benefit of the heart protection outweighs the risk of side effects.

If you're a runner, you could make this analogy: Running on cement sidewalks can make your knees and hips sore from all that pounding. If you do your running in a grassy field, though, the softer surface may be gentler on your legs, causing less pain. However, in the field you run the risk of twisting your foot in a hole or tripping over a hidden object. So which should you do? You have to weigh the benefits versus the risks of each.

> The federal government and the American Heart Association have made it easier for you to decide whether aspirin's benefits are enough to take the risk.

In 2002, the U.S. Preventive Services Task Force—a panel of health experts who evaluate the effectiveness of preventive-health treatments and offer their recommendations for using them—issued guidelines that urged doctors to discuss aspirin with their patients if they have an increased risk of coronary heart disease. The task force found that the benefits offer enough reason to begin aspirin in people with at least a 6 percent chance of having coronary heart disease in the next ten years.

The American Heart Association, however, sets the bar higher: It recommends that aspirin is particularly beneficial for people—if they don't have bleeding disorders or other reasons for avoiding the drug—when their ten-year risk of developing coronary heart disease is 10 percent or higher.

If 1,000 people with a 6 percent risk of coronary heart disease took aspirin, after five years the treatment would prevent one to four "coronary heart disease events," such as nonfatal heart attack, but it would produce up to two cases of bleeding in the brain and two to four cases of major gastrointestinal bleeding.

If 1,000 people with a *10 percent* risk of coronary heart disease took aspirin, it would prevent far more coronary heart disease events— six to twenty—yet the risks of the side effects would remain the same.

For that reason, Dr. Hennekens endorses the recommendation

that people go on aspirin when they have the 10 percent risk. That approach would buy you a much greater chance of preventing a heart attack for the same price of potential side effects.

In women, though, the balance of benefits versus risks may turn out to be different than for men, once more information from research is available, Dr. Buring says. That's because "at any age, a woman has a lower risk of having a heart attack than a man does, but the same risk of an adverse event from taking aspirin," she says.

However, not all experts agree that the perceived useful benefit-risk ratio is enough to warrant healthy people taking aspirin for heart protection, given the evidence currently available. Based on the risk of side effects such as stroke—and a lack of evidence from a number of studies that aspirin reduces the total number of deaths from cardiovascular disease—a panel of experts for the Food and Drug Administration recommended in December 2003 not to allow aspirin manufacturers to recommend the drug for primary prevention on their labeling information.

"There's lots of good evidence that people with heart disease and stroke should take aspirin for secondary prevention. That's sort of written in stone," says William Hiatt, M.D., a panel member and professor and vascular-disease expert at the University of Colorado Health Sciences Center.

However, "Healthy people taking aspirin is, I think, very controversial." The panel's decision would affect "millions of people," and they didn't want to see healthy people taking aspirin long-term, Dr. Hiatt says.

However, the group felt that "some type of primary claim for some group of patients could be developed," according to their meeting notes. Also, they voted unanimously that people should talk to their doctor before beginning aspirin therapy for heart protection.

So be sure to take your concerns and questions about your heart health and aspirin to your doctor. You should only make this decision with your health-care provider after you've discussed your personal level of risk and the benefits that could be awaiting you.

However, you can get a general idea of whether aspirin could help you by using the following measurement tool, called the *Framingham risk score*. This tool was developed using findings from the Framingham Heart Study, which was launched in 1948 to identify risk factors for cardiovascular disease. It has followed residents of Framingham, Massachusetts, and their children for decades—and is now examining yet a third generation of subjects.

The Framingham score is currently the standard in America for measuring cardiovascular risk, says Dr. Lauer of the Cleveland Clinic. Although the Framingham research predominantly used white subjects, this test has been found to be valid in blacks and whites and men and women, he says. It may, however, *over*estimate the risk in Asians and Hispanics.

On the next two pages you'll find the questions for the scoring—the first is for men, the second is for women. Before you begin, you'll need to know your blood pressure, your total cholesterol, and your HDL, or "good" cholesterol. You might also want to use a calculator, although the math involved is simple.

Let's work through a hypothetical person so you'll get the hang of how to figure your score. He's a fifty-three-year-old man with total cholesterol of 210 and HDL cholesterol of 39. So we start by looking in the sections for his age, total cholesterol, and HDL cholesterol, and add 3 + 1 + 1 = 5 points.

He doesn't have diabetes, he smokes, and his blood pressure is 135/87. That gives him another 2 + 1 = 3 points, and added to the 5 points from the first questions gives him a total of 8 points.

Thus, he has a 16 percent chance of having angina, a heart attack, or fatal heart disease in the next ten years, and so his benefit from taking aspirin is likely to outweigh the risks.

If you do begin aspirin therapy to reduce your risk, research has found that taking between 75 and 150 milligrams daily is effective for preventing a first heart attack, says Dr. Kong of Duke University. A low-dose, or "baby" aspirin, contains 81 milligrams.

Again, though, don't make your decision based solely on this chart. Speak to your doctor about whether you should take aspirin, and how much to take. Just because benefits and risks apply in general to large groups of people, they may not apply to you individually as a person. Your doctor can help you decide.

Coronary Disease Risk Prediction Score Sheet for Men
Based on Total Cholesterol Level*

STEP 1

Age

Years	Points	Years	Points
30–34	–1	55–59	4
35–39	0	60–64	5
40–44	1	65–69	6
45–49	2	70–74	7
50–54	3		

STEP 2

Total Cholesterol

(mg/dl)	(mmol/L)	Points
<160	≤4.14	–3
160–199	4.15–5.17	0
200–239	5.18–6.21	1
240–279	6.22–7.24	2
≥280	≥7.25	3

STEP 3

HDL Cholesterol

(mg/dl)	(mmol/L)	Points
<35	≤0.90	2
35–44	0.91–1.16	1
45–49	1.17–1.29	0
50–59	1.30–1.55	0
≥60	≥1.56	–2

STEP 4

Blood Pressure

Systolic (mmHg)	Diastolic (mmHg)				
	<80	80–84	85–89	90–99	≥100
<120	0				
120–129		0 pts			
130–139			1		
140–159				2	
≥160					3 pts

STEP 5

Diabetes

	Points
No	0
Yes	2

STEP 6

Smoker

	Points
No	0
Yes	2

STEP 7 (sum from steps 1–6)

Adding up the points

Age _____
Total Cholesterol _____
HDL Cholesterol _____
Blood Pressure _____
Diabetes _____
Smoker _____
Point Total _____

STEP 8 (determine CHD risk from point total)

CHD Risk

Point Total	10 Yr CHD Risk	Point Total	10 Yr CHD Risk
≤1	2%	7	13%
0	3%	8	16%
1	3%	9	20%
2	4%	10	25%
3	5%	11	31%
4	7%	12	37%
5	8%	13	45%
6	10%	≥14	≥53%

Note: When systolic and diastolic pressures provide different estimates for point scores, use the higher number.

*Information courtesy of National Institute of Health.

Risk estimates were derived from the experience of the NHLBI's Framingham Heart Study, a predominantly Caucasian population in Massachusetts, USA.

(continued)

STEP 9 (compare to man of the same age)

Comparative Risk

Age (years)	Average 10 Yr CHD Risk	Low* 10 Yr CHD Risk
30–34	3%	2%
35–39	5%	3%
40–44	7%	4%

45–49	11%	4%
50–54	14%	6%
55–59	16%	7%
60–64	21%	9%
65–69	25%	11%
70–74	30%	14%

*Low risk was calculated for a man the same age, normal blood pressure, total cholesterol 160–199 mg/dL, HDL cholesterol 45 mg/dL, non-smoker, no diabetes.

Coronary Disease Risk Prediction Score Sheet for Women
Based on Total Cholesterol Level*

STEP 1

Age

Years	Points	Years	Points
30–34	–9	55–59	7
35–39	-4	60–64	8
40–44	0	65–69	8
45–49	3	70–74	8
50–54	6		

STEP 2

Total Cholesterol

(mg/dl)	(mmol/L)	Points
<160	≤4.14	–2
160–199	4.15–5.17	0
200–239	5.18–6.21	1
240–279	6.22–7.24	1
≥280	≥7.25	3

STEP 3

HDL Cholesterol

(mg/dl)	(mmol/L)	Points
<35	≤0.90	5
35–44	0.91–1.16	2
45–49	1.17–1.29	1
50–59	1.30–1.55	0
≥60	≥1.56	–3

Note: When systolic and diastolic pressures provide different estimates for point scores, use the higher number.

Step 4

Blood Pressure

Systolic (mmHg)	Diastolic (mmHg)				
	<80	80–84	85–89	90–99	≥100
<120	-3				
120–129		0 pts			
130–139			0 pts		
140–159				2	
≥160					3 pts

STEP 5

Diabetes

	Points
No	0
Yes	4

STEP 6

Smoker

	Points
No	0
Yes	2

STEP 7 (sum from steps 1–6)

Adding up the points

Age	____
Total Cholesterol	____
HDL Cholesterol	____
Blood Pressure	____
Diabetes	____
Smoker	____
Point Total	____

(continued)

STEP 8 (determine CHD risk from point total)			
CHD Risk			
Point Total	10 Yr CHD Risk	Point Total	10 Yr CHD Risk
≤ 2	1%	8	7%
-1	2%	9	8%
0	2%	10	10%
1	2%	11	11%
2	3%	12	13%
3	3%	13	15%
4	4%	14	18%
5	4%	15	20%
6	5%	≥ 16	≥ 24%
7	6%	≥ 17	≥ 27%

Risk estimates were derived from the experience of the NHLBI's Framingham Heart Study, a predominantly Caucasian population in Massachusetts, USA.

STEP 9 (compare to women of the same age)		
Comparative Risk		
Age (years)	Average 10 Yr CHD Risk	Low* 10 Yr CHD Risk
30–34	<1%	<1%
35–39	1%	<1%
40–44	2%	2%
45–49	5%	3%
50–54	8%	5%
55–59	12%	7%
60–64	12%	8%
65–69	13%	8%
70–74	14%	8%

*Low risk was calculated for a woman the same age, normal blood pressure, total cholesterol 160–199 mg/dL, HDL cholesterol 55 mg/dL, non-smoker, no diabetes.

Why Is Aspirin Measured in Such Odd Doses?

In the United States, you can't find aspirin in dosages containing 50, 75, or 150 milligrams. But you can in Europe.

Instead, in America, you're likely to only find doses containing 81 or 325 milligrams. That's because we still base the aspirin strength on the old-fashioned pharmacy measurements of "grains," says David F. Kong, M.D., a Duke University cardiologist. Ten grains are equal to 648 milligrams, and one grain is equal to 64.8 milligrams.

Thus, a dose you might take for a headache, such as one or two 325-milligram tablets, is equal to 5 or 10 grains (actually, it's a tiny bit more).

A dose you might take for longer-term use, such as preventing a first heart attack, would be 81 milligrams, or 1¼ grains.

Think of it as the difference between measuring in feet and inches versus measuring with metric units—only for aspirin, Dr. Kong suggests.

ASPIRIN AND HEART DISEASE:
PREVENTING ANOTHER HEART ATTACK

If you've already had a heart attack or other serious heart-disease episode, the decision to take aspirin to prevent future problems is much simpler: You should probably be doing it.

"For those who have already had a prior event, the evidence is clear—aspirin has been shown to lower risk of a second event in both men and women," Dr. Buring says.

"If you've already had a heart attack, the risks of taking aspirin are secondary to the risks of having another heart attack, because the number-one risk factor for having another heart attack is having your first heart attack," she says.

Dr. Hennekens recommends aspirin for secondary prevention based on three meta-analyses conducted in 1988, 1994, and 2002. The final one analyzed the results of 287 studies involving more than 200,000 patients who took a variety of medications to reduce blood clotting, most often aspirin.

The people taking aspirin and other anticlotting drugs had a 25 percent smaller risk of nonfatal heart attack, nonfatal stroke (see more about this in chapter 5), and vascular-related death.

However, less than 50 percent of patients with cardiovascular disease are actually taking aspirin to prevent future problems, according to a 1999 study. If more people with cardiovascular disease were using aspirin as recommended, more than 25,000 secondary cardiovascular events could be prevented annually.

The daily dosage that experts typically recommend for preventing additional heart-related problems is 75 to 325 milligrams daily, but again, be sure to talk to your doctor before beginning aspirin therapy.

To be fair, even though this book is about aspirin, another drug commonly used for its antiplatelet effects is clopidogrel (Plavix), and a lot of research attention the past few years has been focused on which works better for heart disease. One such influential study, back in 1996, looked at patients who'd had a recent ischemic stroke or heart attack or had peripheral arterial disease, then followed them for

Could Your Body Be Resistant to Aspirin?

Since more and more people have been taking aspirin for heart protection, researchers have become curious in recent years about a phenomenon called "aspirin resistance."

This term is sometimes used to refer to someone who has a second heart attack despite taking aspirin, and it's sometimes used to describe when aspirin during laboratory tests fails to keep platelets in blood samples from clumping together (which is how it works to prevent heart attacks), says Garret FitzGerald, M.D., a professor of pharmacology and cardiovascular medicine at the University of Pennsylvania.

The number of people who may have aspirin resistance varies widely in the studies measuring it, depending on the definition of the term and the techniques used to examine the platelets. The number ranges from 5 to 45 percent of the general population.

The medical community isn't yet sure about how aspirin resistance can influence your risk of cardiovascular problems, either. Evidence is growing that people whose blood doesn't respond properly to aspirin run a greater risk of health events involving clots, such as heart attacks. But more and larger studies will be needed to shed light on this issue.

Several companies are marketing blood and urine tests to check for aspirin resistance. Dr. FitzGerald thinks it's too early to make a widespread recommendation that people use these tests to influence their aspirin therapy for heart protection.

However, if you have a recurrent heart attack while taking aspirin, your doctor may need to raise your aspirin dosage or put you on a different anticlotting drug.

an average of two years while they took either aspirin or clopidogrel. They then compared the rates of additional ischemic strokes, heart attacks, or vascular-related deaths in the two groups. Clopidogrel reduced the risk of these events by nearly 9 percent more than aspirin.

A later study that only looked at the groups' rate of additional heart attacks found that those taking clopidogrel had a 19 percent smaller risk of a heart attack compared to those taking aspirin.

However, the cost of clopidogrel must be taken into account. A study published in the *New England Journal of Medicine* in 2002 used computer models to compare the cost-effectiveness of the two drugs in preventing cardiovascular events in people with coronary heart disease. According to the authors' estimation, aspirin is more attractive from a cost-effectiveness perspective. Clopidogrel isn't cost-effective unless patients just can't tolerate aspirin for some reason.

OTHER STRATEGIES

Though aspirin may be one way to guard your heart health, it's certainly not the only method you should consider. The National Institutes of Health recommend the following for reducing your risk of heart disease:

- If you smoke, stop. If you don't smoke, don't start.
- Get daily exercise, making sure to check with your doctor first if you're middle-aged or older, have a medical condition, or you've been sedentary. Strive for moderate-intensity aerobic exercise like walking or swimming for at least thirty minutes most days of the week.
- Maintain a healthy weight by following a sensible diet that's low in saturated fat (like that found in red meat and dairy foods) and getting plenty of exercise.
- Keep your cholesterol under control by having it checked regularly; eating a diet high in fruits and vegetables, whole grains, and fish; exercising; and staying at a healthy weight. Your doctor can also prescribe medications to lower your cholesterol if necessary.
- Keep your blood pressure at a healthy level by having it checked regularly; eating a healthy diet, and limiting the amount of sodium you eat; exercising regularly; and avoiding smoking and excessive alcohol use. Your doctor can also prescribe medicines to lower your blood pressure, if necessary.

4

Peripheral Arterial Disease

In 1831, a French veterinarian observed an odd sight on a Parisian street: A carriage horse had developed a limp in its back legs, but the limp only started after a certain period of exertion. After the horse died, the vet did an autopsy on it and found clots in arteries in its legs.

Nearly thirty years later, a prominent Parisian neurologist by the name of Jean Martin Charcot noticed a similar problem in a human patient. This patient wasn't pulling carriages in the street, of course, but rather was a soldier who had been wounded in battle. His injury left him with poor blood flow through arteries going to his legs. Charcot— who was smart enough to have a number of illnesses named after him— remembered the earlier description of the troubled horse and recognized that the same problem was going on in both cases.

That problem is called "intermittent claudication." This is pain in the calf or thigh that flares up after you've walked a certain distance, which may be as short as a block or two. When you stop and rest for five to ten minutes, it subsides. You need roughly the same amount of time after each flareup before the pain goes away.

The claudication, however, is a symptom of a larger problem called peripheral arterial disease, or PAD. And this, in turn, is a sign that unhealthy arteries elsewhere in your body could be setting the stage for even worse problems.

In short, that leg pain could be your body telling you that you should be taking aspirin.

PAD: A WARNING SIGN OF WORSE TO COME

During PAD, blood doesn't flow like it should through the arteries on the outskirts of your body—more specifically, your legs. This is typically the result of the fatty buildup in the arteries known as atherosclerosis. However, not everyone with PAD will develop the symptoms of leg pain.

Research shows that about 12 percent of adults in America will deal with PAD at some point in their lives. The older you get, the more likely you are to have the condition. About one in five people over the age of seventy has it.

> Dr. Charcot didn't know it at the time, but aspirin plays an important role in treating some people with PAD to help them avoid serious—and sometimes fatal—cardiovascular problems.

PAD isn't just a pain in the leg—or the meatier section farther up your backside. If you have the condition, the atherosclerosis that's found in the arteries of your legs may also be elsewhere in your body—including your heart. Even if you've never had a heart attack, your risk of a cardiovascular-related death is similar to the risk in someone with known coronary artery disease.

Cardiovascular disease, in fact, is the most common cause of death in people with PAD. But just because you don't have claudication pain doesn't mean you're free of the condition—up to three-quarters of people with PAD don't have symptoms.

Fortunately, if you have peripheral arterial disease, the long-term use of aspirin can reduce your risk of heart attack and stroke. We'll talk more about specific recommendations for who in particular should consider aspirin, but first let's look at what exactly is going on in the arteries during PAD, so we can understand how aspirin may help.

Aspirin: Helpful for Many People with PAD

Plaque—or debris in the wall of an artery found in atherosclerosis—begins when white blood cells become attracted to the wall of the artery during inflammation. After they migrate into the layer of the artery that's in contact with the bloodstream, they start accumulating fats from the blood. This forms the earliest detectable sign of atherosclerosis called the "fatty streak." Smooth muscle cells accumulate in the site, and calcium also starts to gather.

The plaque eventually contains a fatty core, with a fibrous "cap" on top of it. This plaque juts out into the open space in the blood vessel, slowing blood flow. A clot can form on the plaque, blocking the flow even more.

When this process flares up in your legs, it's likely wreaking havoc in even more crucial blood vessels around your body. According to a paper from a 2003 issue of the *Archives of Internal Medicine,* "The presence of atherosclerotic disease in one vascular bed should not be approached as a localized, isolated disease but as a marker for potentially insidious disease in other vascular regions." Those other vascular regions include the arteries feeding your heart and your brain.

According to the author, roughly half of people with PAD also have coronary artery disease—or plaque in vessels feeding the heart—and up to 40 or 50 percent of people with PAD have also had a diagnosis of cerebrovascular disease, or stroke.

A doctor can easily check you for PAD by comparing the blood pressure in your arms with the pressure in your ankles, using a standard blood pressure cuff and a special device to listen to blood flow in the arteries. Other signs of poor blood flow in your legs include skin redness; hair loss; dry, scaly skin; and brittle toenails.

There's no evidence that aspirin can reduce the symptoms of PAD, such as the leg pain, says William Hiatt, M.D., a professor and vascular-disease expert at the University of Colorado. Nor does it keep the disease from progressing.

However, he says, half the people with PAD should certainly be taking aspirin, and the others *might* get some benefit from it (so long as they don't have a reason not to take it, such as a history of bleeding in the brain).

That's because roughly half the people with PAD also have a history of heart attack or stroke, and aspirin will definitely reduce their risk of more trouble. However, if you have PAD but haven't had a heart attack or a stroke, "I can't give a strong recommendation," Dr. Hiatt says. Aspirin won't reduce your risk of a heart attack in this instance as much as it would if you'd already had one. Also, the FDA declined to approve including the use of aspirin for patients just with PAD on aspirin labeling information.

Plus, another drug called clopidogrel (Plavix) has been shown to be more effective in preventing cardiovascular events in patients with PAD than aspirin. A 1996 study—called the CAPRIE trial—compared the drugs in more than 19,000 people with a history of ischemic stroke, coronary heart disease, or PAD; roughly 6,400 of them had PAD. The people with PAD who took clopidogrel had almost 24 percent fewer cardiovascular events.

In cases where cost is no option, Dr. Hiatt says he'd recommend clopidogrel over aspirin. However, for people without health insurance or drug coverage, cost is likely to be an option.

Many people with peripheral arterial disease aren't using *any* drugs to reduce their risk of clotting, whether aspirin or another drug. In a 2001 study, 40 percent of patients with PAD weren't getting any kind of antiplatelet treatment.

Some experts do feel there's reason for a widespread recommendation for aspirin in patients with peripheral arterial disease. In 2001, the American College of Chest Physicians issued a consensus statement recommending daily aspirin therapy, from 80 to 325 milligrams, for people with intermittent claudication. They also recommend clopidogrel as an alternative option for people with PAD.

OTHER STRATEGIES

Aside from aspirin, a number of lifestyle steps and another medication can reduce the impact of PAD and related cardiovascular problems on your life:

- *Stop smoking.* Smoking is the most important risk factor for developing peripheral arterial disease, and stopping the practice reduces the progression of the disease.
- *Control your diabetes.* If you have diabetes, making sure you keep high blood sugar under control can reduce the chances that you'll develop serious injury to your leg, and it may reduce your risk of heart attack.
- *Keep blood pressure under control.* Keeping your blood pressure reined in can reduce your risk of stroke.
- *Exercise.* Many studies have shown that regular exercise will allow you to walk farther without leg pain. You'll get the greatest improvement from exercising at least thirty minutes at least three times weekly. Be sure to talk to your doctor before starting an exercise program.
- *Consider another medication.* A drug called cilostazol (Pletal) is FDA-approved for claudication, and it may allow you to walk farther without leg pain. This drug isn't for use in people with heart failure, though.

Section III

Protecting Your Brain

You've now learned how aspirin can keep one of your most vital organs—your heart—ticking along. Now it's time to turn to an even more important organ: your brain.

Aspirin can help keep your brain healthy through much the same process as it helps your heart, by keeping it well-nourished with blood. Keeping an adequate blood supply helps protect you from strokes and the decrease in mental abilities that may follow them.

Aspirin's anti-inflammatory power may also help protect you from Alzheimer's disease, which can rob you of your memories and your ability to think normally.

5

Strokes

The days after World War I were disastrous for the health of President Woodrow Wilson—and they weren't too happy for the pharmaceutical company that had brought aspirin to the world twenty years earlier, either.

Wilson took off to Paris after the conclusion of the war to help negotiate a peace treaty. His life had frequently been interrupted by illness; he'd been diagnosed with arteriosclerosis—or hardening of the arteries—and he may have had more than one stroke before he became president. He was also prone to health breakdowns during times of stress.

After two trips to France and a grueling effort to sell his ideas on the treaty and the League of Nations to a skeptical Senate, Wilson stubbornly took off on a train tour to promote his ideas directly to the American people. On September 23, 1919, he stumbled through a speech in Pueblo, Colorado. He had an apparent stroke after the train pulled out of town.

After returning to Washington, he had a *major* stroke, leaving him paralyzed on one side. His close aides kept Wilson's cabinet in the dark about the severity of the president's illness for months while he slowly recuperated. He eventually regained the ability to maintain some of his official duties, but remained emotionally and physically impaired.

At the same time, Bayer, aspirin's developer, was having its own health crisis stemming from the war.

In late 1918, the U.S. government auctioned off Bayer's American holdings, including their patents and trademarks. A West Virginia firm bought the assets for $5.3 million and started making its own Bayer aspirin in America.

It's possible that Woodrow Wilson had taken aspirin, since he was also plagued with headaches throughout his life. But no one knew at the time that regularly taking the drug might have helped reduce the risk of the kind of strokes that felled him.

But nearly a century later, doctors have plenty of reasons to think that aspirin can be an important tool in helping you live a longer, fuller, stroke-free life.

Your Brain: A Thinking Machine That Needs Lots of Fuel

Your brain is one hungry customer, and if its supply of food is interrupted, even briefly, the results can be catastrophic to your health.

This is what happens during a stroke, which strikes more than 700,000 Americans each year. About 160,000 people die of stroke-related causes annually, and two-thirds of those who survive a stroke will suffer some sort of brain impairment afterward.

Doctors can only offer a small handful of drugs to lessen your risk of having a stroke, and aspirin is one of them. It's not perfect for every person—and some people should definitely avoid it. However, it should be a "first-line treatment" in most people who've had a stroke, and you should consider taking it if you *haven't* had a stroke but your risk of having one is high, says David Tong, M.D., an associate neurology professor and associate director of the Stanford Stroke Center at Stanford University in Palo Alto, California.

Dr. Tong once wrote an editorial in a medical journal that asked "Can aspirin ever be surpassed for stroke prevention?" Given its price compared to other drugs with a similar method of reducing your risk, it'll be tough, he says: "It's virtually impossible to beat it, because its cost is so low it's basically free."

Aspirin can help your brain through the same mechanism as it helps your heart—by keeping the blood flowing to it.

Every heartbeat brings your brain another serving of fuel, in the form of vital oxygen and glucose. The brain consumes a whopping 20 percent of the oxygen used by your body when it's at rest. Though most of the tissues in your body can go without oxygen for several minutes if the need arises, your brain can only go without oxygen for a few seconds. If the oxygen-bearing blood flow to your brain totally stops for only ten seconds, you'll lose consciousness.

Though your brain only weighs about three pounds—accounting for about 2 percent of an average person's total weight—it receives about 20 percent of the blood your heart pumps out. Each minute, three-quarters of a liter of blood flows through your brain. That adds up to 285 gallons of blood coursing through your noggin each day.

Your brain requires this oxygen to convert glucose into energy. Glucose, which is also known as blood sugar, is the only substance that your brain uses to produce energy. However, your brain needs to convert the glucose to a substance called ATP before using it for energy, and this process requires oxygen.

Since your brain has no way of storing up energy to use for later—and even at rest it requires as much energy as a 20-watt lightbulb—it needs a constant supply of glucose and oxygen. During a stroke, however, the flow of blood halts to part of your brain. Depending on which area is deprived, the damage from the interruption can kill you, leave you disabled, take away your ability to speak, or rob you of other faculties.

A number of risk factors increase your odds of having a stroke, some you can change and some you can't.

Having high blood pressure is the most potent risk factor for

Act Quickly If You May Be Having a Stroke

According to the American Stroke Association, the following warning signs of a stroke should prompt you to call 911 immediately:

- Sudden numbness or weakness in your face, arms, or legs—particularly if it's on one side of your body.
- Sudden confusion, or trouble speaking or understanding what's going on around you.
- Sudden vision loss in one or both eyes.
- Sudden dizziness, loss of coordination, or difficulty walking.
- Sudden severe headache and you don't know what's causing it.

stroke, according to the American Stroke Association. The higher your blood pressure, the higher your risk of stroke. Since this condition is silent, you probably won't even know you have it unless you have your blood pressure checked. Fortunately, high blood pressure is treatable.

Smoking is also a changeable risk factor; the habit reduces oxygen in your blood and makes you more likely to have clots. Having high cholesterol or diabetes and being sedentary or obese also raise your risk of stroke.

The risk factors that increase your odds of stroke that you *can't* change include your age and your race. People become more likely to have a stroke as they grow older. African Americans are twice as likely to have a stroke or die of stroke or its complications as other racial or ethnic groups in America.

Also, if you've had a heart attack your odds of stroke go up. And if you've already had a stroke, your risk of having another goes *way* up.

Although aspirin can help protect you from strokes in much the same way it guards against heart attacks and heart disease—by making your blood less likely to clot—this isn't necessarily as helpful in strokes as heart disease. Compared to the process that causes heart disease, which follows a similar course in most people, the causes of strokes are more varied from person to person, says Mitchell Elkind, M.D., M.S., an assistant professor of neurology at Columbia University in New York, who has studied aspirin in stroke prevention.

Also, there are two kinds of strokes, one of which is much more common than the other. Aspirin can be useful in preventing the more common type, but it can actually make the less common type of stroke even *worse*. So you and your doctor must give extra thought to your particular situation before putting aspirin to work for you.

How the Blood Flows to the Brain— and What Can Stop It

Your brain's blood supply travels up to the organ from the heart via two sets of arteries: Your *carotid arteries* and your *vertebrobasilar* arteries.

The carotid (pronounced cah-ROT-ted) arteries provide the majority of the blood to your brain. You have a carotid artery on each side of your neck, and each forks into the internal and external carotids. The internal carotids carry blood to the brain, and the external carotids carry blood elsewhere in your head.

The vertebral arteries—one on each side of your body—branch off arteries that pass under your collarbones. The vertebral arteries then run up your neck next to your vertebrae, or bones in your spine, then join together under your brain to form the basilar artery.

All these arteries supply blood to an elaborate network of branches of blood vessels that course through the brain. We could name them, but it would take all day.

During a stroke, the blood flow to brain cells is interrupted

Aspirin Lends a Hand in High-tech Treatments

If an artery in your neck isn't supplying your brain with enough blood, you may need an operation to remove the blockage—called carotid endarterectomy—or push it aside to let the blood through to prevent a stroke. But this may loosen emboli in the artery that can *cause* a stroke!

Fortunately, aspirin—either alone or in combination with another drug—can help protect you during and after the procedure.

Doctors commonly give patients aspirin before an endarterectomy to make blood less likely to clot, reducing the risk of a stroke. A 2004 study from England found that also giving the patients clopidogrel (Plavix)—a drug that also reduces platelet clotting in the blood through a different mechanism—greatly reduces the risk of developing multiple emboli versus aspirin alone.

A newer type of procedure for opening blocked carotids, which is becoming more common, can also be safer with aspirin. During carotid stenting, doctors place a stent—or wire-mesh tube—into the blocked area to prop it open, allowing blood to flow through. Though surgeons use a filter during the procedure to catch loosened chunks of material so they don't get to the brain, clots that are loosened during the procedure or that form on the stent afterward are still a concern.

A 2001 study by researchers from the Cleveland Clinic Foundation in Ohio in the (ominously named) *Journal of Invasive Cardiology* found that the combination of aspirin and clopidogrel given for thirty days after a stent installation was associated with a low rate of ischemic events, such as a stroke, transient ischemic attack, or heart attack.

through one of two ways. The most common type of stroke—an *ischemic stroke*—occurs when an artery becomes blocked and not enough blood can get through. These account for about 80 percent of stroke cases.

The other 20 percent or so are cases of *hemorrhagic stroke*. These are caused by a blood vessel that ruptures, spilling blood into the brain. Either can be deadly, but hemorrhagic strokes tend to be worse. And aspirin plays far different roles in each. Let's take a closer look.

The Aspirin Vocabulary

- *Anticoagulant.* A type of drug that prevents clots. Warfarin (Coumadin) is an anticoagulant, and it prevents clotting by minimizing other substances your blood needs to form clots.
- *Antiplatelet.* A drug that prevents blood clots from forming by keeping platelets in your blood from joining together. Examples include aspirin, clopidogrel (Plavix), and ticlopidine (Ticlid)
- *Atherosclerosis.* The process in which plaques made of fat, cholesterol, and other materials accumulate in an artery wall. Clots can form on plaques, or pieces of plaque can get caught in the bloodstream, either of which can cause a stroke.
- *Embolus.* A blockage in an artery that comes from somewhere else in the body. This can be a blood clot or piece of plaque. When an embolus blocks the flow of blood, the interruption is called an *embolism.*
- *Hemorrhagic stroke.* A less-common cause of stroke, these are caused by ruptured blood vessels on the surface of the brain or deep in the organ. This robs brain cells of their blood supply, and the escaped fluid also can damage surrounding brain cells by increasing pressure on them.
- *Ischemic stroke.* This results when something blocks an artery that brings blood to the brain. The blockage may be a blood clot that forms on a buildup of plaque in the artery, or it may be a clot or piece of material carried in the bloodstream from elsewhere in the body.
- *Thrombus.* A blood clot.
- *Transient ischemic attack.* Also called a TIA or a "mini-stroke," this is a temporary interruption of blood to your brain cells. Symptoms go away completely in less than twenty-four hours. It may be caused by a blood clot or embolus lodged in a vessel that dissolves on its own, allowing blood flow to return.

Ischemic Strokes

The word ischemic simply means "insufficient blood flow." The same malfunctions in your arteries that contribute to heart attacks can also contribute to these. A plaque accumulates in the wall of an artery and protrudes out into the bloodstream. This lowers the flow of blood in the artery on the other side of the plaque, like when a stream is partially dammed.

These plaques tend to grow in arteries in spots where the direction of the blood flow changes, such as where vessels branch off or make a sharp curve. These areas of prime real estate for plaques occur at a number of spots in the neck and brain, such as where the vertebral artery branches off the artery that feeds it, or where the internal and external carotid arteries part ways.

A blood clot, also called a *thrombus,* can form on a plaque and completely halt blood flow through the artery where the plaque has already slowed the flow.

Another type of ischemic stroke can arise from an *embolus.* This is a chunk of debris that becomes caught up in the current of the bloodstream and becomes lodged in an artery. An embolus is often a blood clot, but it can also be a chunk of material that breaks loose from a plaque and gets swept away in the bloodstream. What defines it, though, is that it originates from some other part of the body than where it halts and causes the problem. When an embolus becomes wedged in an artery, it's called an *embolism.*

Emboli (the plural of embolus) can be created in the heart, and these often arise from a mishap known as *atrial fibrillation* (AF). In this condition, the atria, or upper chambers of the heart, don't contract smoothly and strongly—instead, they quiver irregularly. As a result, blood becomes stagnant in the atria and forms clots in the nooks and crannies of the chambers. A clot can then get caught up in the blood flow and travel out of the heart toward other organs. It may travel to your brain until it hits a vessel that's too small for it to continue.

Aspirin Is Proper Treatment for Many with Atrial Fibrillation

Because atrial fibrillation may arise months to years before a stroke, and it's treatable with aspirin and other medications, most strokes associated with AF are potentially preventable.

Warfarin (Coumadin) is a prescription anticoagulant that makes your blood less likely to clot. It's been found to reduce your risk of stroke if you have AF by about 68 percent. Aspirin isn't as powerful; it only reduces the risk by about 20 percent. However, warfarin is more expensive, and its benefits must be balanced by the risk it poses of bleeding complications and the added effort that your doctor must make to regularly monitor your dosage to make sure that it's working properly.

As a result, organizations like the American Heart Association (AHA) and the American College of Chest Physicians (ACCP) believe that aspirin is the appropriate choice for people with atrial fibrillation who are at low or moderate risk of ischemic stroke, with warfarin reserved as a bigger weapon for people at higher risk.

According to the ACCP, you should take 325 milligrams of aspirin daily if you have AF and are sixty-five or younger with no other risk factors. You can take this dose of aspirin, or move to warfarin, if you're sixty-five to seventy-five or have diabetes or coronary artery disease. If you're over seventy-five or have a history of stroke, TIA or embolus, high blood pressure, several types of heart-valve problems, or more than one intermediate risk (diabetes or coronary artery disease, or being sixty-five to seventy-five), you would move to the high-risk category treated with warfarin.

AF can go unnoticed, as it may cause no symptoms. However, it may bring a sensation that your heart is racing, and you may feel light-headed and short of breath. It may only occur every once in a while, or it may come and go for a few hours. If you think you're having episodes of AF, talk to your doctor, who can diagnose the condition by hooking you up to a monitor to check the electrical activity of your heart.

About 2.4 million Americans have atrial fibrillation, and this number is expected to more than double by 2040 as the population gets older. As many as 15 percent of strokes in the United States happen to people with AF.

Once a plaque, clot, or embolus cuts down the blood flow enough to cause an ischemic stroke, the brain tissue affected by the lack of blood will quickly begin to die. How you're affected depends on where the damaged brain cells are located and how widespread the damage is.

President Wilson's stroke was said to be caused by a thrombosis that killed cells in the right side of his brain.

A condition that's similar to an ischemic stroke but is less serious is called a *transient ischemic attack,* or TIA. These are caused by an obstruction in a vessel that blocks the blood flow briefly, but goes away on its own. Symptoms of a TIA include weakness and numbness on one side of the body, loss of vision, and difficulty remembering words—but these typically last less than a few hours, and the TIA leaves no permanent impairment. However, a TIA is an important sign that a serious stroke could strike you soon and requires medical attention.

Aspirin's main role in preventing ischemic stroke is to keep platelets in the blood from sticking together to form a clot, so blood continues to flow past narrowed spots in the arteries feeding the brain.

Hemorrhagic Strokes

This is where using aspirin for preventing and treating strokes becomes complicated. During hemorrhagic strokes—which are much less common than ischemic strokes—an artery ruptures, unleashing its flow deep into the surrounding brain tissue or into the small area between the surface of the brain and the skull.

As the leaked blood presses outward, something has to give to accommodate the extra pressure. Since your bony skull won't expand, the blood may instead push aside and destroy surrounding brain tissue. The rise in pressure can also put the pinch on other arteries in the brain, slowing their blood flow to other parts.

Symptoms of a hemorrhagic stroke usually appear quickly, and these events aren't preceded by smaller warning strokes, like the TIAs that can come before ischemic strokes. However, sometimes people who are having a hemorrhage have a terrible headache.

Hemorrhagic strokes are more often fatal and cause a poorer outcome in general than ischemic strokes. You definitely want to avoid them if you can.

Unfortunately, large studies have shown that taking aspirin can cause a slight increase in a person's chance of having a hemorrhagic stroke. According to the U.S. Preventive Services Task Force, if 1,000 people took aspirin for five years, it would cause up to two additional hemorrhagic strokes. That might not sound like much of a risk—unless you turn out to have one of those two strokes.

HOW TO USE ASPIRIN
IF YOU'VE NEVER HAD A STROKE

If you've never had a stroke, heart attack, or cardiovascular disease, there's not much scientific evidence to suggest that you should start taking aspirin to prevent a possible stroke.

"Most strokes are ischemic and aspirin probably protects us against those. But at the same time it *does* slightly increase the risk of having a hemorrhagic stroke. The Physicians' Health Study determined that aspirin will reduce the risk of a heart attack even in healthy individuals who haven't had a first event. But it's not so clear that's the case for stroke," Dr. Elkind says. "In terms of someone (healthy) going into the office of their primary care doctor and saying 'Hey, shouldn't I be on an aspirin to prevent a stroke?' the answer would be no."

However, once your risk factors for stroke start adding up, your doctor may act quickly to get you on aspirin, Dr. Tong says. "We give aspirin at the drop of a hat if a patient has any significant risk factor for vascular disease; anyone (with) hypertension, cholesterol, smoking, or diabetes, they pretty much automatically get aspirin—even for primary prevention." These risk factors may make aspirin even more important for you as you grow older and get into age groups that bear a heavier stroke risk.

Aspirin May Save Your Vision

A condition that's commonly considered by eye doctors to be "the prime medical emergency in ophthalmology" is likely an ailment you've never heard of. But if you do develop it, a familiar drug—aspirin—can reduce your risk of blindness.

The condition is called temporal arteritis, also known as giant-cell arteritis. It's an inflammation of the temporal artery, which runs over your temples between your ears and the outer corner of your eyes, as well as blood vessels coming off the external carotid arteries. The disease is almost always found only in people over the age of fifty; and about 50 percent of people with the condition also have an ailment called polymyalgia rheumatica, which brings stiffness in the hips and shoulders.

Symptoms of temporal arteritis include scalp sensitivity, a throbbing headache on one side of the head, blurry or reduced vision, and jaw pain. Complications of temporal arteritis include blindness—usually irreversible—due to lack of blood flow to the eye's optic nerve or retina, as well as stroke.

The standard treatment for it is corticosteroid drugs, says Stephen Paget, M.D., a professor of medicine at Weill Medical College of Cornell University in Ithaca, New York, who studies the condition. However, research has shown that "patients treated with aspirin as opposed to just steroids alone have a much lower incidence of visual loss and other central nervous system problems such as stroke," he says.

Adding aspirin to steroid therapy "adds an extra dimension" of control of the clotting and blockage in the blood vessels that occurs on the inflammation on the vessel wall, Dr. Paget says.

If you read the chapter on aspirin and your heart, you learned how to calculate your risk of developing heart disease in the next ten years, then use the results to help decide with your doctor whether the benefits of aspirin outweigh your risk.

A similar quiz for determining your stroke risk is also available and was also devised using data from the Framingham Heart Study, which has tracked the health of generations of residents of a Massachusetts town. It's not used as often since heart disease is more common than stroke, and it's not been proven to be as valid a predictor as the heart-disease tool, Dr. Elkind says. However, you can use it to get a sense of your risk of having a stroke, he says, which you can then discuss with your doctor.

It's designed for people who are fifty-five and older and includes separate scoring sheets for men and women. On these two pages you'll see the information for men, and on the following two pages the information for women.

Let's go through the worksheet using a hypothetical woman, to learn how the scoring system works.

Score Your Stroke Risk for the Next Ten Years—Men*

BOX A

Points	0	+1	+2	+3	+4	+5	+6	+7	+8	+9	+10
Age	55–56	57–59	60–62	63–65	66–68	69–72	73–75	76–78	79–81	83–84	85
Systolic blood pressure—untreated	97–105	106–115	116–125	126–135	136–145	146–155	156–165	166–175	176–185	186–195	196–205
Systolic blood pressure—treated	97–105	106–112	113–117	118–123	124–129	130–135	136–142	143–150	151–161	162–176	177–205
Diabetes	No	Yes									
Cigarettes	No		Yes								
Cardiovascular disease	No				Yes						
History of atrial fibrillation	No				Yes						
Diagnosis of left ventricular hypertrophy	No					Yes					

BOX B

Your Points	10-year probability	Your Points	10-year probability	Your Points	10-year probability
1	3%	11	11%	21	42%
2	3%	12	13%	22	47%
3	4%	13	15%	23	52%
4	4%	14	17%	24	57%
5	5%	15	20%	25	63%
6	5%	16	22%	26	68%
7	6%	17	26%	27	74%
8	7%	18	29%	28	79%
9	8%	19	33%	29	84%
10	10%	20	37%	30	88%

BOX C

Compare with your age group	Average 10-year probability of stroke
55–59	5.9%
60–64	7.8%
65–69	11.0%
70–74	13.7%
75–79	18.0%
80–84	22.3%

*Information courtesy of National Institutes of Health.

Score Your Stroke Risk for the Next Ten Years—Women*

BOX A

Points	0	+1	+2	+3	+4	+5	+6	+7	+8	+9	+10
Age	55–56	57–59	60–62	63–64	65–67	68–70	71–73	74–76	77–78	79–81	82–84
Systolic blood pressure—untreated		95–106	107–118	119–130	131–143	144–155	156–167	168–180	181–192	193–204	205–216
Systolic blood pressure—treated		95–106	107–113	114–119	120–125	126–131	132–139	140–148	149–160	161–204	205–216
Diabetes	No			Yes							
Cigarettes	No			Yes							
Cardiovascular disease	No		Yes								
History of atrial fibrillation	No						Yes				
Diagnosis of left ventricular hypertrophy	No				Yes						

BOX B

Your Points	10-year probability	Your Points	10-year probability	Your Points	10-year probability
1	1%	10	6%	19	32%
2	1%	11	8%	20	37%
3	2%	12	9%	21	43%
4	2%	13	11%	22	50%
5	2%	14	13%	23	57%
6	3%	15	16%	24	64%
7	4%	16	19%	25	71%
8	4%	17	23%	26	78%
9	5%	18	27%	27	84%

BOX C	
Compare with your age group	**Average 10-year probability of stroke**
55–59	3.0%
60–64	4.7%
65–69	7.2%
70–74	10.9%
75–79	15.5%
80–84	23.9%

*Information courtesy of National Institutes of Health.

She's fifty-seven years old, and her systolic blood pressure (the top number) is 132, even though she's taking medication for high blood pressure. She has diabetes, but no history of cardiovascular disease, and she smokes. She has no history of atrial fibrillation or left ventricular hypertrophy, which is thickening of the walls in one of the heart's chambers, which can be caused by high blood pressure.

She gets one point for her age, six points for her blood pressure, and three points for her diabetes. She picks up another three points because she smokes, giving her a total of thirteen points. As shown in Box B, thirteen points means she has an 11 percent risk of having a stroke in the next ten years. In Box C, we see that women in her age group have only a 3 percent risk of stroke on average, which means our sample woman has a much higher risk. Whether or not she's a good candidate for aspirin should be decided with her physician's help, but it's something she should discuss with her doctor.

USING ASPIRIN IF YOU HAVE
HAD A STROKE OR HEART DISEASE

Once you've had a stroke, the decision whether to take aspirin gets much easier—you probably should be on it, unless your stroke was hemorrhagic. If you've had a hemorrhage, it's unlikely that you'd want a drug that helps you bleed more freely. Doctors can identify what kind of stroke a person has had "virtually 100 percent of the time" by using a CAT scan shortly after the event, Dr. Elkind says.

"Once somebody has had a first event, then they're considered at high risk of having *another* event. Obviously if it was a hemorrhagic stroke, they wouldn't be on aspirin or another blood-thinning agent because of the propensity to bleed again. But for ischemic strokes, which are the majority, just about everybody should be on aspirin or another blood-thinning agent for the rest of their lives," he says.

If you're treated immediately after a stroke, daily aspirin can reduce your risk of an additional stroke in the next few weeks by a quarter, according to an analysis of two major studies that looked at nearly 40,000 patients. In one of the studies, people took 160 milligrams of aspirin daily for a month and in the other, people took 300 milligrams daily for two weeks.

According to these results, if a group of one thousand people started taking aspirin within forty-eight hours of an ischemic stroke, they'd have seven fewer recurrent ischemic strokes and four fewer deaths by other causes, but they'd have two more hemorrhagic strokes. This means nine people would be saved from life-changing (or ending) events, simply by taking aspirin.

The benefits of taking aspirin don't just protect you in the few weeks after a stroke—they can reduce your risk in the long-term, too.

Taking regular aspirin will make you about 13 percent less likely to have a recurrent ischemic stroke, says Dr. Tong, the Stanford University neurologist.

You might be thinking that a 13 percent reduction in risk doesn't seem like much protection for something that experts consider a wonder drug. But, as Dr. Tong points out, the other blood-thinning drugs available don't offer you much more protection.

"Even though that sounds like a small benefit, what else do we have?" he asks. Several other anticlotting agents besides aspirin are considered good first-line drugs to use to reduce the risk of additional ischemic strokes, but whether they're better or not is a controversial matter, he says.

A major study from 1996 compared the use of aspirin for three years versus clopidogrel (Plavix) in more than 19,000 people who'd had an ischemic stroke, heart attack, or peripheral arterial disease. It found that clopidogrel was about 9 percent better than aspirin at reducing the risk of another ischemic stroke or heart attack, or vascular-related death.

This, however, just means that Plavix will reduce your risk of ischemic stroke by about 14 percent, compared to aspirin's 13 percent, Dr. Tong points out.

A 2001 study that compared aspirin to the blood thinner warfarin (Coumadin) in more than 2,200 patients who'd had ischemic strokes that didn't involve emboli from the heart found that the more expensive drug offered "no additional benefit over aspirin in preventing recurrent ischemic stroke" in these people. The authors concluded that "aspirin, either alone or in combination with some other antiplatelet agents, appears to be a well-justified choice for the prevention of recurrent ischemic stroke."

However, combining aspirin with other antiplatelet agents is controversial. Since combining these drugs can increase the risk of severe bleeding, using them in this way may not be a good thing for stroke prevention. Plus, Coumadin should only be used for stroke prevention in special circumstances.

A 2003 study compared the effectiveness of aspirin with the drug ticlopidine (Ticlid) in African Americans—a group with an extra-heavy burden of stroke—who'd had an ischemic stroke that didn't involve emboli from the heart. After two years of follow-up, the study found no statistically significant difference in the drugs' ability to prevent additional strokes or vascular-related death. "We regard aspirin as a better treatment for aspirin-tolerant black patients" with a history of this sort of ischemic stroke, the authors noted.

Where aspirin gains a significant advantage over these other drugs, in Dr. Tong's viewpoint, is its price.

A year's worth of 81-milligram aspirin, a dosage recommended for stroke prevention, would cost you about $12 or less. A year's worth of Plavix would cost you about $1,320, according to an online pharmacy. A year's worth of Ticlid would cost about $859.

"From a pharmacoeconomic perspective, it's very difficult to beat it," Dr. Tong says. To beat it, "You'd have to have a medicine that was basically extremely potent and not cause bleeding complications, or you'd have to have a medicine that's as inexpensive as aspirin, and that won't be easy."

The exact dose that is necessary to prevent strokes has changed in recent years, he says—with expert opinions shifting from high doses to low doses and, among some experts, back to high doses. In general, 81 to 325 milligrams daily is thought to be acceptable in offering protection, he says.

If you do have another stroke when you're already taking aspirin, your doctor may choose to increase your aspirin dosage or switch you to another of the drugs that work to reduce blood clots, says Dr. Elkind, the Columbia University neurologist.

OTHER STRATEGIES

If you're interested in reducing your chances of a stroke, you can do a lot more in addition to taking aspirin. Here are some suggestions from the American Stroke Association and the National Institutes of Health:

- Keep your blood pressure in the normal range. Steps to lower it include keeping a healthy weight; eating a diet lower in sodium and higher in potassium; exercising regularly; and taking blood pressure medications if your doctor recommends them.
- Avoid smoking.
- Exercise regularly and eat a healthy diet, even if you don't have high blood pressure.
- If you have diabetes, work to keep it under control.
- Try to keep your stress level down.

6

Alzheimer's and Vascular Dementia

Auguste was fifty-one years old, and her mental health was deteriorating.

She grew jealous over her husband's activities and feared that people wanted to kill her. She constantly moved the furniture around their apartment. Her memory loss grew worse and worse, and so did her screaming. She eventually had to be placed in an institution, where she would spend the few remaining years of her life.

The year was 1901, and the location was Frankfurt, Germany. Just two years before, Bayer had trademarked its drug Aspirin, which chemist Felix Hoffmann had figured out how to make in a laboratory less than two hundred miles away.

Life didn't get any easier for Auguste in the mental asylum. She didn't understand what was going on around her and feared that the doctors wanted to harm her. She didn't always make sense when she spoke and couldn't keep track of the time or where she was. She would drag her blankets around, screaming and screaming. She eventually grew confined to her bed and died on April 6, 1906.

The doctor who checked her into the asylum had moved on, but requested to examine her brain after she died, since he was interested in brain structures and diseases. He found that her brain was shrunken and riddled with clumps and tangles of material, and many neurons— or brain cells—were missing.

That November, the doctor—whose name was Alois Alzheimer, by the way—presented his findings of Auguste's case to a convention of German psychiatrists. In 1910, a colleague authored a psychiatry textbook in which he gave a name to a particular form of dementia. He called it *Alzheimer's disease.*

The condition didn't generate much interest from the public or researchers during Dr. Alzheimer's lifetime, or for decades afterward. When he was examining Auguste's brain, relatively few people lived to an age when the disease becomes common, so it appeared unusual. It was only in the late 1970s that scientific interest in the condition exploded, paving the way for it to become a household name.

Recent research has given experts good reason to think that aspirin may help make a person less likely to develop not only Alzheimer's disease, but also another brain disorder that causes confusion and difficulty doing normal tasks called *vascular dementia.* Let's take a closer look at these conditions, then move on to how aspirin and related drugs can play a beneficial role.

The aspirin vocabulary

- *Beta-amyloid plaques.* Chunks of protein found in the brain outside the neurons. These are found in people without dementia, but are found in greater amounts in people with Alzheimer's.
- *Cerebral cortex.* A thin layer of "gray matter" covering your cerebrum—which is the large, upper part of the brain divided into

the left and right hemispheres. Your cerebral cortex is responsible for your higher mental abilities, your behaviors, and other important functions.

- *Glia.* These cells, which vastly outnumber neurons in your brain, support and nourish the neurons.
- *Infarct.* An area of dead tissue caused by lack of blood flow to the area, usually from a blood clot or other blockage in an artery.
- *Neurofibrillary tangles.* Another sign of Alzheimer's, these are tangled bits of proteins found inside neurons; they contribute to the death of the cell.
- *Neurons.* Also known as "nerve cells," these send signals to one another while you're thinking, sensing the world around you, and moving.
- *Tau.* The type of protein involved in neurofibrillary tangles.
- *Vascular dementia.* A decrease in mental abilities caused by a series of small strokes. It affects some mental functions but not others in a pattern that makes it distinguishable from Alzheimer's disease. Also called multi-infarct dementia.

DEMENTIA: A PROBLEM AFFECTING EVER-GROWING NUMBERS OF PEOPLE

The term "dementia" refers to a group of symptoms related to unclear thinking that can stem from a number of brain disorders. The long list of mental deficits that can be involved in dementia include:

- Memory loss
- Difficulty concentrating
- Confusion
- Difficulty learning, calculating, and thinking abstractly
- Trouble understanding speech and forming words
- Mood changes, including irritability
- Lack of ability to care for oneself
- Lack of interest in normal activities

Although it's common for folks to become a little forgetful as they journey through their senior years, dementia *isn't* a normal part of aging. It's a sign that something has gone wrong in the brain.

Often, that something is Alzheimer's disease, the most common cause of dementia. According to the National Institute on Aging, up to four million Americans may have the condition. Though it seldom occurs before the age of sixty, it becomes more common with advancing age. Nearly half the people who live past the age of eighty-five may have it. After symptoms arise, people live, on average, another eight years.

The number of people with the condition has more than doubled since 1980, and with the Baby Boomer population growing grayer, up to sixteen million people could have it by 2050, according to the Alzheimer's Association.

However, if a treatment could be found that could delay the onset of the disease by only five years, it could cut the number of people with Alzheimer's nearly in half after fifty years, according to the association.

After Alzheimer's disease, the second most common form of dementia is vascular dementia, which refers to symptoms caused by insufficient blood flow to the brain. This condition is also sometimes called *multi-infarct dementia,* which is actually a common cause of vascular dementia. An *infarct* is an area of dead tissue caused by lack of blood flow (you may remember from chapter 3 that another name for a heart attack is a myocardial *infarction,* referring to the dead heart muscle that ensues).

Multi-infarct dementia (MID) can be the result of lack of blood flow to parts of the brain caused by strokes, which result in dead spots of brain tissue. A person with Alzheimer's disease shows gradual symptoms that slowly and steadily grow worse. People with MID, by contrast, will more likely have sudden mental changes that slowly improve, or at least stabilize. Their symptoms may again take a turn for the worse when they have future strokes or other incidents resulting in decreased blood to the brain.

WHAT ALZHEIMER'S LOOKS LIKE
UNDER THE MICROSCOPE

When people have Alzheimer's, not only do their mental abilities change, but so does the physical appearance of their brains.

If you've seen a normal brain—perhaps in a jar in a museum—you know that it is covered with large grooves that give it its "squiggly" appearance. These grooves are called *sulci,* which is plural for sulcus. In a person with Alzheimer's, the brain shrinks, and these sulci become wider.

The normal brain also has open pockets inside called ventricles, which are filled with cerebrospinal fluid. These ventricles share the fluid with the spinal cord (this is the fluid the doctor samples during a "spinal tap"). During Alzheimer's, these ventricles grow larger as brain tissue shrinks.

Much of the shrinkage occurs in the *cerebral cortex.* This is the surface of the cerebral hemispheres, which form the bulk of the brain, and it's what you probably picture when you think of "the brain." The cerebral cortex is grayish in color, and it's composed of billions of nerve cells, called *neurons,* and other cells, called *glia.* The neurons are the cells that transmit messages to each other like electricity through wiring. Neurons help you see and hear and help send messages to your body that make it move. Glia are cells that nourish, support, and protect the neurons. You have perhaps nine times more glial cells in your head than neurons, though the neurons do the thinking.

Your cerebral cortex, though only about as thick as the cover on a hardback book, handles most of the information processing in your brain. Damage found in Alzheimer's disease often affects the parts of the brain that handle memory, reasoning, planning, and reading.

Brain shrinkage isn't the only problem seen in Alzheimer's disease. The condition is also marked by scattered, abnormal structures called *beta-amyloid plaques* and *neurofibrillary tangles.* These are the bits of material that Dr. Alzheimer found in Auguste's brain one hundred years ago.

Plaques are dense chunks of protein and cell matter that are found outside of neurons. Beta-amyloid is made of snippets of a larger protein that actually seems to be useful in helping repair damaged neurons. For some reason, pieces of beta-amyloid begin joining together, along with other substances, to form plaques. These plaques are found around the cerebral cortex, as well as in a structure deeper in the brain called the hippocampus, which plays a role in memory storage.

The neurofibrillary tangles are found inside the neurons. They're composed of a type of protein—called *tau*—that gives support to structures called microtubules inside the neuron, which help carry nutrients within the cell. For some reason, the bits of tau become attached and tangled up with each other. This causes the microtubules to fall apart, which may cause the neuron to have difficulty communicating with other neurons and later to die.

Though many healthy older people have some plaques and tangles in their brains, people with Alzheimer's disease have many more. Experts don't know if the plaques are a cause of the disease, or merely an effect of it, but these plaques may be related to inflammation in the brain.

Substances involved in inflammation have been found in the plaques. Whether this inflammation is helpful, in allowing the brain to deal with the plaque formation, or harmful, in contributing to neuron death, is still up in the air, according to the National Institutes of Health.

However, research has found that the betaamyloid protein may cause damage that your body then responds to with inflammation. This inflammation may then cause more beta-amyloid to be produced, starting a vicious cycle.

Another familiar substance has been found in the brains of people with Alzheimer's: the COX enzyme. As you'll see throughout this book, this enzyme plays a role, or suspected role, in heart disease, stroke, and cancer. The enzyme is vital for the production of prostaglandins, which are multipurpose chemicals that help protect organs such as your stomach, but also are involved in harmful inflammation. COX comes in at least two types—COX-1, which is always present throughout your body, and COX-2, which pops up more at sites of inflammation.

Giulio Pasinetti, M.D., Ph.D., a professor of psychiatry, geriatrics, and neuroscience at the Mount Sinai School of Medicine in New York, has conducted research that showed a link between excess COX and prostaglandin in the brain with more beta-amyloid.

"There is also evidence suggesting that anti-inflammatory drugs might also by themselves be able to actually block beta-amyloid generation," he says. However, blocking the creation of this substance would require concentrations of the drug in the body equivalent to taking forty painkillers a day.

Elevated COX-2 has been found in neurons in the hippocampi of people with Alzheimer's, and it's been found to be correlated with the withering of neurons and the density of plaques in the region.

Another reason why researchers think inflammation may be connected to Alzheimer's is because nonsteroidal anti-inflammatory drugs (NSAIDs)—a family that includes aspirin—seem to reduce a person's risk of developing the disease. We'll talk more about that later; let's first look at another leading cause of dementia that might be preventable with aspirin.

VASCULAR DEMENTIA: A DIFFERENT SORT OF LOSS

Vascular dementia is responsible for about 20 percent of the cases of dementia in America, making it the second-leading cause. It can result from hemorrhages, which are leaks from blood vessels in the brain, or from ischemia, in which an area of the brain doesn't receive blood because a vessel becomes blocked by a blood clot or other piece of material. Strokes aren't required to cause vascular dementia—it can even come from poor blood flow due to partially blocked vessels serving the brain, says Gustavo Roman, M.D., a professor, neurologist, and vascular-dementia expert at the University of Texas Health Science Center in San Antonio.

The signs of vascular dementia are noticeably different from Alzheimer's, at least to the trained eye. Vascular dementia (also called VaD) can begin suddenly, then follow a step-wise pattern of worsening after each new event that brings lack of blood to the brain. Also, unlike Alzheimer's, VaD doesn't typically bring early and severe memory loss, nor the early impairments in speaking and calculating ability.

People with VaD typically have severe early losses in "executive function," which are abilities involved in organizing one's life, such as the ability to make plans and shift between actions. These problems aren't seen so early on during Alzheimer's. Finally, people with VaD usually have trouble with their gait and shuffle when they walk. That's not usually a problem in people with Alzheimer's until late in the disease.

People with VaD also usually have a history of strokes, transient ischemic attacks (or "mini-strokes"), and hypertension. In people over the age of sixty-four, research has found that 25 to 33 percent have dementia after an ischemic stroke. Factors that increase the risk of dementia after a stroke include older age, smoking, severe or recurrent strokes, and complications of the stroke including seizures and pneumonia caused by inhaling stomach contents.

It's possible for a person to have both vascular dementia and Alzheimer's disease, and the former can worsen the latter. Studies have shown that people who've had one or two strokes require fewer plaques and tangles in their brains before they show signs of dementia. And vascular disease in older patients with Alzheimer's may make their dementia obvious earlier.

As you learned in the previous chapter, regular aspirin use may help make a person less likely to have an ischemic stroke. This may be because it makes blood less likely to form clots, and by decreasing inflammation that contributes to accumulation of plaque in the arteries.

In the next sections, we'll look at the research that shows why aspirin might be helpful for these conditions.

Aspirin and Other NSAIDs: Supporting Evidence in Alzheimer's

Scientists have proposed a number of theories on how inflammation can cause damage in Alzheimer's, and how aspirin and other NSAIDs may offer protection.

The COX-2 enzyme might produce free radicals—or rogue oxygen molecules—inside neurons that could damage the cells. The prosta-glandins that the COX enzymes help produce may also increase the effects of a neurotransmitter called glutamate. Neurotransmitters are chemicals that neurons send between each other to "talk" to each other, and some neurons use glutamate. If too much glutamate lingers in the space between neurons, it can overstimulate cells, causing them to die. Thus, inhibiting the COX enzymes inhibits the prostaglandins, which could reduce this overstimulation with glutamate.

To consider whether high- or low-dose aspirin might help protect against Alzheimer's disease, a Swedish study from 2003 looked at 702 people age eighty and older and measured their use of aspirin. There was a "significant" association between the use of high-dose aspirin and a lower frequency of Alzheimer's disease, and the aspirin users had better-preserved mental abilities, too.

An Italian study from 2003 looked at more than 2,700 seniors, with an average age of seventy-seven, who were enrolled in home-care programs. The study found that those who took NSAIDs had almost a 50 percent lower risk of having Alzheimer's.

Closer to home, a 2002 study that followed elderly residents of Cache County, Utah, found that longer use of NSAIDs provided a greater reduction in risk of Alzheimer's. Former NSAID users showed substantially fewer new cases of the disease, leading the researchers to conclude that "long-term NSAID use may reduce the risk of Alzheimer's disease, provided such use occurs well before the onset of dementia. More recent exposure seems to offer little protection."

This finding that aspirin or other NSAIDs only work to reduce the risk of Alzheimer's disease when they're taken years before the disease would strike is typical, Dr. Pasinetti says.

Clinical studies—which have provided people with anti-inflammatory drugs rather than observed how they used them on their own—have failed to show the same results that the drugs are helpful in preventing the disease, he says. This may be because the drugs in these studies have usually been given for too short a period and too late to prevent the disease.

More information on the ability of NSAIDs to reduce the risk of this disease may be provided by a study launched in 2001, which will follow roughly 2,600 seniors with a family history of Alzheimer's-like dementia for seven years. They'll take either naproxen sodium (Aleve), which is an over-the-counter NSAID; celecoxib (Celebrex), which is a prescription COX-2 inhibitor; or a placebo.

Vascular Dementia: Supporting Evidence for Aspirin

Fewer studies have been conducted linking aspirin with a lower risk of vascular dementia.

However, "the more strokes you have, the more likely you will have loss of cognition, loss of independence, and dementia," Dr. Roman says. Aspirin can help prevent recurrent ischemic strokes, thus lowering your risk of having more of these events that can rob you of your mental abilities.

Even if you haven't had a stroke, but your hypertension or high cholesterol puts you at high risk for one, taking aspirin before you ever have a stroke may help keep you dementia-free.

Only in recent years have big studies for stroke and heart attack prevention included a cognitive test to show mental functioning as an "endpoint," or event of interest, Dr. Roman says. However, researchers have shown that treating people for hypertension—a major risk factor for stroke—appears to make them less likely to develop dementia compared to people given placebo.

At the time this chapter was being written, a team of Australian researchers was embarking on a five-year study to give low-dose aspirin or a placebo to 15,000 people age seventy and over, to see if the drug reduces the risk of vascular dementia and major cardiovascular events.

In explaining why they were launching the study, the researchers pointed to research showing that aspirin reduces the risk of nonfatal stroke in middle-aged subjects and should do the same in elderly people. Aspirin's anti-inflammatory abilities may also help reduce plaque formation in arteries, cutting down on events that bring lack of blood flow to the brain, they say.

Quoting earlier research, the lead researcher of the Australian study, Dr. Mark Nelson, of Monash University in Victoria, points out that 22 percent of people in their late sixties from a group of 3,658 older people were found to have small infarct-like injuries in their brains. These areas of damage were associated with a history of stroke and hypertension and poor cognitive ability.

It's reasonable to suspect that these areas of damage are caused by small blockages in blood vessels, which regular aspirin therapy might help prevent, he adds.

OTHER STRATEGIES

Doctors don't know enough about aspirin's effect on dementia to recommend it yet. However, taking a few other simple steps may help keep your mind sharp:

- Reduce your risk of stroke by having your doctor check your blood pressure regularly. Keep your high blood pressure controlled by taking appropriate medications, following a low-salt diet, and keeping a healthy weight. Regular exercise is helpful, too.
- Keep your mind busy by playing games, working puzzles, and staying socially active.

Section IV

Protecting You from Cancer

It's a word that can strike fear into the strongest of hearts. But unfortunately, many people will have to deal with cancer at some point in their lives.

Doctors can offer a wide variety of surgeries, medications, and other treatments to banish cancer from our bodies and allow us to live for years afterward. However, these procedures can be disfiguring and extremely unpleasant to endure. Preventing the disease from ever striking is a far more appealing option.

And aspirin might be an important part of a cancer-prevention plan. Doctors have found that the simple, easily available drug may help reduce a person's risk of developing cancer at many sites around the body. In this section, you'll learn the latest evidence that aspirin may help prevent cancer in the digestive tract, the breast, and many other body parts.

7

Digestive Cancers

In the mid-1800s, a pioneering German physician named Rudolph Virchow concluded that there was a link between inflammation in the body and cancer development.

Virchow was a pathologist—an expert who inspects tissues for diseases—who left a lasting mark on the field. He coined the term *ischemia*, which is a lack of oxygen to cells that occurs in heart attacks and some strokes, and named a number of tumors.

He also observed in tumors some of the same cells and substances that are found in inflamed tissue, leading him to believe that cancer may begin at sites that are chronically inflamed. However, the scientific community was skeptical, since few experts felt that a healthy process like inflammation—the way the body defends itself against infection and injuries—could cause such a dreadful disease.

Fast-forward to Colorado in the late 1970s. William Waddell, a surgeon at the University of Colorado Medical School, was treating a family with a condition called "familial adenomatous polyposis," called FAP for short. It's a hereditary condition that causes people to develop hundreds of polyps in their colon at an early age. These growths— called *adenomatous polyps*—can turn into colorectal cancer in anyone, but in people with FAP, at least one polyp starts turning cancerous around age twenty, according to the American Cancer Society.

One of Dr. Waddell's patients had an abdominal tumor, and the physician thought that inflammation might be a cause of it. He prescribed a medication called sulindac (Clinoril), which is a nonsteroidal anti-inflammatory drug (NSAID). Aspirin is also an NSAID.

The drug didn't have an impressive effect on the tumor, but it noticeably improved the polyps in the patient's rectum. The drug turned out to also be helpful in treating several of the patient's relatives with the disease, too.

Though Dr. Waddell's work was based on a hunch he had, rather than his scientific research, it represented a bridge from using anti-inflammatory drugs to reduce the number of tumors in lab rats and mice to using the drugs in humans, says Michael Thun, M.D., the vice president of epidemiology at the American Cancer Society, who has been studying aspirin's effects on cancer for more than a decade.

In the 1970s, scientists found that certain tumors in animals had concentrated amounts of prostaglandins, which are hormones with a variety of effects in the body, both good and bad.

They were curious whether blocking these prostaglandins with aspirin would inhibit the development of tumors. So the scientists exposed mice and rats to carcinogens, then gave them aspirin and aspirin-like drugs, and as they'd suspected, "Many studies over more than ten years consistently showed that a variety of aspirin-like drugs would do that (inhibit tumors)," Dr. Thun says.

Later on, in 1991, a medical journal published a paper linking aspirin use with a decreased risk of colorectal cancer, but "the study was met with skepticism," Dr. Thun says.

The next year, Dr. Thun and colleagues submitted a paper to the *New England Journal of Medicine,* documenting research in which they combed through data on hundreds of thousands of people to examine their use of aspirin and their rate of death from colorectal cancer. They found an inverse relationship between the two; in other words, taking aspirin was associated with a smaller risk of having fatal cancer.

The idea still seemed too novel, and the journal wanted more evidence before they'd publish the paper. The researchers found enough other studies hinting at aspirin's use in cancer "to make this seem plausible," Dr. Thun recalls.

The paper attracted a huge amount of attention and drew scientific interest and funding to research the links between aspirin and other anti-inflammatory drugs and cancer prevention.

Experts now have plenty of reasons to believe that these drugs can prevent a variety of cancers by decreasing inflammation. The bulk of the work examining aspirin's effects against cancer has been done on colorectal cancer, where the evidence is particularly strong that the drug is helpful. But it also may help make a person less likely to develop cancer of the esophagus, stomach, breast, lung, prostate, and other organs.

> **One of Dr. Thun's grandparents is from Wuppertal, Germany—the city where chemist Felix Hoffmann made his aspirin discovery. It's a small world.**

"I think it's exciting that a drug like aspirin seems to be effective in preventing colon cancer," says Andrew Chan, M.D., M.P.H., a Harvard Medical School instructor and staff gastroenterologist at Massachusetts General Hospital, whose research focuses on ways to prevent colon cancer with medications.

It's too early yet to make sweeping recommendations that people should take aspirin to prevent cancer, say Dr. Chan, Dr. Thun, and other experts you'll be meeting in the coming pages. But, Dr. Chan says, it's certainly encouraging to have evidence that a readily available medication can help prevent a condition as serious as cancer.

Aspirin may someday prove to be a useful tool for *some* people to reduce their risk, or it may become a useful member of a cancer-preventing team when combined with other protective strategies, he says. In addition, understanding how aspirin affects the disease will give doctors deeper insight into how the disease begins and progresses, which in turn may point them toward other anticancer medications.

"I think there's many different ways this can go, and each of these ways is potentially very exciting," Dr. Chan says.

This chapter will highlight the exciting new discoveries that offer evidence that aspirin might provide some protective effects against cancers in the digestive tract—specifically, the colon and rectum, esophagus, and stomach. The following chapters in this section will cover the tantalizing hints that aspirin may be helpful against cancer in the breast and elsewhere in the body.

COLON CANCER

First, let's take a look at what colon cancer is, and where it comes from.

Your Colon in Health and Illness

Your colon, also known as your large intestine, is found at the lower end of your digestive system. This organ—about five feet in length—receives processed food that your small intestine didn't absorb and draws water and minerals it contains back into your body. The final portion of the colon is the rectum, which temporarily holds stools until you can find a restroom.

The Aspirin Vocabulary

- *Adenocarcinoma.* These are cancers arising from cells in the lining of your colon, stomach, and rectum. They make up more than 95 percent of colorectal cancers.
- *Adenoma.* A growth arising from the surface of the colon that's also known as a polyp. Though most adenomas won't turn into cancer, almost all colon cancers are thought to come from adenomas. Larger polyps are more likely to turn into cancer.
- *Angiogenesis.* The creation of new blood vessels, such as those formed to feed nutrients to a growing tumor.
- *Apoptosis.* The process in which cells self-destruct because they're

---

too damaged to function properly or they've reached their preset time limit.

- *Epithelium.* A thin layer of cells that covers your skin and lines the inner surfaces of organs throughout your body, including your esophagus, intestines, and bladder. Cancers that develop on epithelial surfaces are called *carcinomas,* and they account for more than 80 percent of all cancers.
- *Free radicals.* These are rogue molecules that can cause damage in your body, including damage to the genes that keep cells behaving normally.
- *Metastasis.* When cancer cells spread to other parts of your body, like through your bloodstream or lymph system.
- *Mutation.* An alteration in a gene that can cause a cell to behave abnormally, perhaps by dividing at an excessive rate or refusing to die.
- *Observational study.* A type of study in which the researchers merely observe what subjects are doing, but don't control any behaviors.
- *Randomized controlled study.* A study in which the researchers control an activity they're trying to measure, such as giving aspirin to people rather than merely asking them if they take it or not. The "random" aspect helps ensure that similar types of people are put into different categories being compared.

Colorectal cancer, which is cancer arising in the colon and rectum, is the third most common cancer in American men and women, according to the ACS. About 150,000 cases were diagnosed in 2004; roughly 70 percent of these were colon cancer, and the rest were cancer of the rectum.

Colorectal cancer accounts for 10 percent of all cancer deaths. African Americans are hit particularly hard; their death rate from the disease is roughly 30 percent higher than whites', and more than twice as high than in Asians and Hispanics.

These growths are almost always a form of cancer called *adenocarcinoma*. And most of these, in turn, are thought to come from polyps called *adenomas* (also known as adenomatous polyps). These are what people with FAP develop in great numbers.

However, in most people, for the most part, these polyps don't develop into cancer. In fact, roughly one-third of adults over the age of fifty have these fleshy, bulbous growths in their large intestine. Plus when a polyp does turn bad, it's not as if it suddenly decides to become a villain. Experts think that it takes about ten years for a polyp to develop and turn into cancer.

The symptoms that indicate that you may have a polyp include blood in your stool or on the toilet paper after you use the restroom, or increased diarrhea or constipation. Your doctor can check for polyps in your rectum by feeling around in the area with a gloved finger and by having a sample of your stool tested for blood. Other ways of detecting polyps include taking an X-ray of your colon after you've had an enema containing a substance called barium, which makes the polyps easier to find. Or a physician can examine your colon with a viewing device in procedures called a flexible sigmoidoscopy or a colonoscopy, and remove any growths he or she finds to test them for cancer.

Don't Forget to Check for Polyps!

Once you blow out the candles on your fiftieth birthday cake, it's time to start a new tradition: Making sure you have a healthy colon.

At fifty, you should start one of these testing methods, according to the American Cancer Society: a fecal occult blood test, which checks a stool sample for blood, every year; a flexible sigmoidoscopy, which allows a doctor to inspect your rectum and part of your colon, every five years; a yearly fecal occult blood test *and* a flexible sigmoidoscopy every five years; a double-contrast barium enema every five years; or a colonoscopy, which allows the doctor to view your entire colon, every ten years.

You should start being screened more often, starting at a younger age, if your risk of colorectal cancer is particularly high. This includes people who have already had colorectal cancer or adenomas; occurrence of these conditions in a parent, sibling, or child under the age of sixty (or more than one of these relatives at any age); a history of inflammatory bowel disease; or a family history of FAP or hereditary colon cancer.

Polyps are an important development on the road between healthy intestine and cancer. But the role of inflammation in the disease is getting a lot of attention these days from experts, too.

People with inflammatory bowel disease (IBD), like people with FAP, are at increased risk of developing colon cancer.

IBD is actually an umbrella term that encompasses two conditions—Crohn's disease and ulcerative colitis. In each disease, the body's immune system attacks the digestive tract, causing it to become inflamed and marked with ulcers. Crohn's disease can strike anywhere in the digestive system, from the mouth to the other end—though it generally affects the intestines. Ulcerative colitis, as its name implies, only affects the colon. Symptoms of either condition include bleeding and diarrhea.

More is known about the link between ulcerative colitis and cancer, but Crohn's disease is thought to increase the risk, too. Once a person has ulcerative colitis for eight years or so, the risk of cancer begins rising. After that, the risk goes up by about ½ to 1 percent each year; the more area in the colon that's affected by the disease, the greater the risk of cancer.

We'll take a closer look shortly at exactly how both inflammation and cancer develop in a moment, but here's how they interact in people with IBD.

Inflammation in the colon may play a number of roles in encouraging normal cells to turn cancerous. For one thing, the inflammation generates *free radicals,* which are rogue molecules that are missing electrons. They try to alleviate the shortage by zipping around your body trying to grab electrons from other molecules. These free radicals can cause damage to the genetic material in colon cells that are responsible for maintaining regular, orderly turnover in these cells.

Take, for example, a gene called the p53 gene. It is responsible for keeping tumors suppressed by telling cells to die when their DNA becomes damaged. If this gene becomes *mutated,* or altered, by free radicals, the change may help allow cancerous cells to grow into tumors.

Inflammation in the cells lining the colon also speeds up the natural process by which these cells are created and die off. This increased turnover in cells helps set the stage for cancer.

A player in the development of colon cancer during inflammation is the COX-2 enzyme. As you learned earlier in this book, an enzyme called COX is necessary to produce prostaglandins in your body, which are substances that can have both helpful and harmful effects on your health. The COX comes in at least two forms; COX-1 is thought to have a "housekeeping" function that protects your body, while COX-2 generally shows up more during harmful inflammation and cancer. Aspirin inhibits both types.

The normal colon lining doesn't produce COX-2, but the enzyme is found in areas of inflamed colon lining in people with ulcerative colitis, and it's also found in even larger amounts in polyps and colon cancer. The enzyme can indirectly produce free radicals and also spur the growth of new blood vessels that feed nutrients to cancerous cells.

Inflammation: A Good Idea . . . When It Doesn't Go Too Far

Inflammation may sound like a process that you'd *never* want to go on in your body. Why would redness, swelling, heat, and pain ever be a good idea?

Actually, inflammation is an important process designed to protect your body from harmful elements and keep it working properly. Inflammation kicks in to minimize the damage from a variety of threats, from splinters to sprained ankles to infections.

When your tissues are injured, cells release substances called *mediators,* including prostaglandins and histamine. These create all sorts of changes in the area. Blood vessels in the region become wider, allowing more blood to flow to the injury. This creates the warmth and redness you feel and see and allows more cells in your immune system to rush in and get to work.

Some mediators allow the blood vessels to become more permeable, allowing white blood cells from your immune system, as well as other products, to seep through the vessels into the injured site. The flow of fluid and other substances from your bloodstream into the area causes swelling, which in turn puts pressure on pain receptors and causes pain. While you might not enjoy the pain or disability in an injured body part, they're useful in keeping you from, say, walking farther on a sprained ankle and causing more damage to it.

Proteins in the blood that leak into the injured area form clots, which help wall off the injury or infection, therefore inhibiting the damage from spreading out farther in your body. Different types of white blood cells show up to the scene in stages, where they start cleaning up the area by eating bacteria, dead cells, or other things that don't belong there. The pus you may see at sites of infection is actually fluid mixed with spent white blood cells and other debris from the battlefield.

Your body's inflammatory defenses don't just occur at isolated spots, though: They can also encompass your whole body. The invader that triggers the inflammatory mediators can also bring on a fever. The higher temperature in your body helps kill or slow down disease-causing germs, and it may help rev up your immune system, too.

All told, the process of inflammation makes a nice watchdog against intruders and troublemakers. But what happens when the watchdog starts barking all night for no apparent reason? What if it stops patiently waiting to bite burglars and instead starts chomping on your own leg?

Sometimes inflammation can rage on for long periods of time when the problem it's attacking is particularly persistent. And sometimes the inflammation isn't even confronting an actual threat. This can be a problem because the effects of the inflammation can cause serious damage to your body . . . like cancer.

Inflammation in response to the *H. pylori* bacterium—the bug that causes ulcers—is linked to stomach cancer. Some hepatitis viruses are connected to liver cancer. Inflammation in your lungs due to irritating chemicals from smoking or from breathing in asbestos is linked to lung cancer. Stomach acid rising into the throat—called reflux—can set the stage for esophageal cancer, and irritation from gallstones can help lead to cancer of the gallbladder.

We'll look at exactly how inflammation might play a role in colorectal cancer development, and how aspirin can reduce the risk—but first let's look at how cancer begins and takes hold in your body.

Cancer: When Cells Break the Rules and Go Wild

Your seventy-five trillion or so cells are normally good citizens, longing to follow the rules for the greater good of the community—in this instance, your body.

Cells reproduce through a process called *mitosis.* In short, this means that a cell splits in two, and both new cells contain the same genetic material as the original. Each of these splits in two, and so forth.

Cells form new cells when needed, like to replace old and damaged cells, or to ramp up for challenges, like when new mothers require larger milk-producing glands in their breasts to feed a baby, and cells in the glands multiply rapidly to meet the need.

They also normally die off quietly and without complaint when they can no longer function properly or they reach their preordained time limit. This is called *apoptosis.* You won't remember this, but it happened to you when you were an embryo in the womb and cells in your hands died off, leaving you with individual fingers instead of webbed paddles.

Sometimes, though, cells start acting in their own self-interest and grow in an uncontrolled manner due to *mutations,* or alterations in the DNA they contain that gives them instructions on how to reproduce and grow.

For example, the little recorded genetic message to a cell telling it when to die might become mutated. So the cell doesn't know when it should die, and after it divides, then *two* cells don't know when to die. One of these cells might also develop another mutation that orders it to multiply uncontrollably. Thus, *it* divides and forms more and more cells, all of which also have the mutation that keeps them from going through apoptosis, or regularly scheduled death. Another mutation might allow one of these cells to influence blood-vessel growth to feed a growing tumor—a process called angiogenesis, which deprives normal cells of their nutrients.

Smoking can cause these sorts of mutations, and so can many chemicals. Radiation from the sun or X-rays can cause mutations in your genetic material. So can some viruses. And you can inherit mutations that lead to cancer from your parents.

Considering the mind-bogglingly huge number of times that your cells will reproduce in your lifetime, it's not surprising that mutations frequently occur. In fact, you have about a million mutations each day! It's a scary thought. However, just because you develop a mutated cell doesn't mean it will turn into a tumor. Fortunately, your immune system's job is to take out these cells that are acting in an unsavory manner.

Also, cells need to go through several mutations—perhaps up to seven—before they can go completely bonkers, and cancerous cells also must win space in your body to grow and a food source before they can thrive.

The Story Behind the Cancer Sign and Constellation

If you were born in late June through late July, you may have wondered why your zodiac sign is named after the dreaded disease cancer. If you know the night sky, you might have also wondered why a constellation is called Cancer.

It all comes down to crabs. A crab represents the zodiac sign of Cancer, and also supposedly is found in the constellation. The Latin word for crab is "cancer."

When you look at a cancer under a microscope, it appears to have legs branching out into the surrounding area, making it resemble a crab. By comparison, a tumor that's benign, or noncancerous, is typically encased in a smooth capsule.

Most cancers in humans start on epithelial surfaces, which are sheets of cells lining your mouth and many organs, like your lungs, stomach, bladder, and intestines. Once a growing mass of irregular cells grows deeper and breaks through the *basement membrane* below the epithelium, the trouble really starts. The cancer can *metastasize,* or spread to other parts of the body, in the bloodstream or through lymph channels.

Inflammation can contribute to cancer in many different ways and many different stages. It can damage cells' DNA. It can make cells resistant to apoptosis, and it can stimulate angiogenesis to improve blood supply to sites. Cancer cells can also be the target of your body's inflammation, but instead of fighting the cancer, the inflammation actually helps it develop further.

"Cancer results from the promiscuous activity of different molecular pathways that have gone awry, a process that's set in motion by some genetic insult," says Jaye Viner, M.D., M.P.H., the program director of the gastroenterology and other cancers research group in the division of cancer prevention at the National Cancer Institute. That means that if doctors want to figure out how to prevent cancer, they have an awful lot of contributing factors they need to investigate and target, and a number of critical steps along the way they may need to interrupt.

One of the players that's attracted a lot of attention with its "promiscuous activity" is the COX enzyme, which is where aspirin comes into play as an ally in the fight against cancer.

The COX-2 enzyme is found in higher amounts in about 85 percent of colorectal cancers, says Raymond DuBois, M.D., Ph.D., a professor of cancer biology at Vanderbilt University School of Medicine in Nashville, Tennessee. It's also found in higher levels in other types of tumors, such as in the colon, esophagus, lung, prostate, skin, breast, and bladder.

Many of these tumors also produce more prostaglandins than their surrounding tissue (remember that COX is necessary in producing prostaglandins). Researchers have found that knocking out the COX-2 in lab rodents by manipulating their genes reduced intestinal tumors in the animals.

COX can make cells resistant to dying when they're supposed to do so, and the prostaglandins can help support a cancer's ability to grow and metastasize, Dr. DuBois says.

Aspirin or other NSAIDs, however, disable COX, therefore cutting down on production of prostaglandins, which researchers believe may be a benefit of aspirin in cancer prevention. Besides its effect on the COX enzyme, aspirin may also affect cancer development through "other parallel pathways that are just now becoming unraveled," Dr. DuBois says.

Aspirin and other NSAIDs are appealing because they may offer a way to interrupt the process long before a damaged cell becomes a cancer cell, Dr. Viner says.

"From a cancer prevention perspective, the target of these drugs is actually the process, rather than the resulting cancer. The process of carcinogenesis (cancer development) is generally regarded as what happens up until the point that cells invade into the basement membrane," she says. "Once you get to a full-blown cancer state, I don't think anyone's arguing that an NSAID alone will put cancer at bay," she says.

Halting growths before they invade into the basement membrane is "really a critical juncture, because at that point the cells have the potential to metastasize. That really puts patients in a much more vulnerable state. In the vast majority of cases, the lethality of cancer is not simply because you're developing a mass, it's because that mass has invaded key structures or has metastasized to the lung, the liver, the brain, or wherever, and is causing problems that way."

Another reason to concentrate on cancer prevention, which aspirin might offer, is that a tumor may already have a billion cells before your doctor can detect it. At that point, you may be facing disfiguring surgery, or harsh chemotherapy and radiation to get rid of the cancer—which may or may not work.

Doesn't popping an aspirin sound more appealing?

The Science Supporting Aspirin for Colorectal Cancer

Early research exploring the effects of NSAIDs on colorectal cancer used mice. It's possible to breed mice with a mutation that causes them to develop polyps that turn into cancer, making them a small-scale model for humans' disease.

"The nice thing was that we learned that commonly used drugs—aspirin and other NSAIDs—got to the target," Dr. Viner says. So scientists started giving aspirin and other anti-inflammatory drugs to the animals to prove their potential to prevent cancers.

In the early 1990s, research started looking at whether human populations who took aspirin and other anti-inflammatory drugs had fewer colorectal polyps and cancers. Plenty of studies showed that people who used aspirin and other NSAIDs had fewer polyps, fewer colorectal cancers, and less death from colorectal cancer, she says.

"This was an extremely solid premise for moving forward, having the animal data, having a strong hypothesis, and then having the observational human data. Also this slew of studies showed consistent effects across ages, genders, and geographies . . . the overwhelming majority of data pointed to the fact that something important was going on, even though a lot of the basic work had not been entirely worked out yet," Dr. Viner says.

For example, a number of studies throughout the 1990s and early 2000s associated aspirin use with a 40 to 50 percent reduction in colon cancer.

However, observational studies—which are those that simply look at people's behaviors and try to connect it with a change in their health—are "subject to a number of different uncertainties, biases, and limitations," says John Baron, M.D., M.S., M.Sc., an epidemiologist and professor of medicine at Dartmouth Medical School in Hanover, New Hampshire.

People might not correctly tell the investigators how much aspirin they take and how often. Or people who take aspirin may also generally exercise more, eat differently, or be better educated than people who don't take aspirin, which can influence their cancer risk, he says. It's a challenge to "untangle the web of influences" and ensure that investigators take these variables—called confounding factors—into account.

However, Dr. Baron and other researchers have more recently added discoveries to the wealth of knowledge on aspirin and cancer that come from studies called randomized controlled studies. In these, the researchers control factors—such as giving aspirin to subjects— rather than just observing whether they occur or not. These have been called the "gold standard" of clinical studies, and they can offer the best evidence that one factor actually causes another—such as aspirin reducing the risk of colorectal cancer.

These studies examine aspirin's effect on *polyps* rather than its effect on colorectal cancer. That's because colon cancers take so long to develop, and the odds of any given person getting colorectal cancer are slim—thus researchers would have to include a large number of people in such a study and watch them for a long time. They can get results on polyps more quickly and inexpensively. Plus, reducing the number of polyps in patients will presumably reduce the number of colorectal cancers.

In one of these studies, reported in the *New England Journal of Medicine* in 2003, Dr. Baron and colleagues gave groups of roughly 370 people a daily dose of either 81 milligrams or 325 milligrams of aspirin, or a placebo pill with no effect, for three years. Neither the patients nor the researchers knew who was getting what. All the people had had polyps removed previously, but were shown to be polyp-free when the study began. After three years or so, they had another colonoscopy to see how many growths they had.

People taking the 81-milligram aspirin wound up having 19 percent fewer polyps than people in the placebo group. People taking 325 milligrams had four percent fewer. The researchers concluded that aspirin had a "modest effect" in reducing polyps. Why the lower dose showed a greater effect is odd; perhaps you only need a certain amount of aspirin to protect you, which both offered, and the difference in effect was just a random occurrence.

Another study, reported in the same issue of the journal and led by Robert Sandler, M.D., M.P.H., of the University of North Carolina in Chapel Hill, looked at 635 patients who'd had previous colorectal cancer. Half took 325 milligrams of aspirin a day and half took a placebo. After roughly a year, each underwent a colonoscopy so a doctor could check for polyps.

The results were more impressive. In fact, a board of people who were monitoring the study's safety requested that it be terminated early due to the benefits seen in people taking aspirin. People in the aspirin group had a 35 percent lower risk of polyps than the people taking a placebo. Plus it took longer for polyps to show up in those taking the aspirin.

Just how high of a dose of aspirin people would need to take to prevent colon cancer is still up in the air. Dr. Chan—the Harvard instructor who commented earlier in the chapter—led a study published in 2004 looking into this question.

They looked at data from more than 27,000 women on their use of aspirin and their history of colon polyps. Not surprisingly, the researchers found that taking aspirin reduced the risk of polyps. However, the greatest amount of protection was in the women taking more than fourteen aspirins a week. The harmful effects of this much aspirin—including digestive damage and possible bleeding in the brain—may outweigh the possible benefits.

The Choice: Should You Take Aspirin to Reduce Colon Cancer?

In the heart disease and stroke chapters, you found charts to help determine whether your risk of developing one of these diseases was worrisome enough to warrant taking aspirin regularly. However, that kind of guidance isn't available for cancer yet, since experts don't know as much about aspirin's effects on the disease to know if the possible benefits outweigh the risks.

A large number of people would need to take aspirin for years for a small number of them to enjoy more life without colorectal cancer, Dr. Baron points out. When that many people are taking aspirin, a rare side effect—say, a 1 in 10,000 chance of having fatal gastrointestinal bleeding, for example—starts piling up. Doctors want to make sure that enough benefit will come from the cancer prevention to warrant the complications.

At some point, doctors will likely have an algorithm, or formula, for calculating whether someone's risk of cancer is great enough to warrant taking aspirin to reduce the risk, says Dr. Thun of the American Cancer Society. A formula someday may even incorporate your cardiovascular risk into a formula with your cancer risk; "There's tremendous interest in working toward that," Dr. Thun says.

Still, aspirin looks appealing now. Dr. Sandler wrote an editorial accompanying Dr. Chan's study when it was published in the *Annals of*

Internal Medicine. In it, he wrote that "If we had a pill that could prevent cancer, we might escape the need for potentially disfiguring surgery or toxic chemotherapy. If the pill were familiar, cheap, and readily available, so much the better."

However, until more information comes along on whom to use it for, aspirin should only be considered a *possible* option for preventing the disease in people with a higher risk for adenomas, like people who've had colon cancer or some other aspect in their personal or family history that would put them at special risk. People taking it should also never have had ulcers or bleeding in the brain if they want to take aspirin to prevent colon cancer, Dr. Sandler writes.

Aspirin shouldn't take the place of having regular checkups to see whether you have polyps, he points out. However, aspirin could make colonoscopies easier and safer for you by causing a decrease in adenomas for your doctor to have to inspect or remove.

The potential benefits emerging from aspirin's possible use in preventing colon cancer aren't limited to just aspirin. Scientists might also use what they know about aspirin's effects on cancer to develop safer versions of the drug—or find that drugs that work in a similar fashion as aspirin may be a "viable option for patients to use to prevent cancer," Dr. Chan says.

One of those drugs might be COX-2 selective inhibitors. However, in September 2004, executives at Merck, the company that makes Vioxx, a COX-2 inhibitor, announced it was stopping sales of the product after researchers investigating long-term use of the drug to prevent colon polyps discovered an unacceptably high risk of heart attacks and strokes. In late 2004, it's unknown if and when the drug will return, and how the increased scrutiny will affect other COX-2 inhibitors.

Aspirin may also someday prove to be particularly helpful when it's combined with other cancer-preventing drugs that protect against different processes that are involved in cancer development. The effect of this combination could be greater than the effect of each agent alone, "allowing us to use lower and safer doses of each drug," Dr. Viner says.

ESOPHAGEAL CANCER

Heartburn is an aggravating problem that can turn your enjoyment of a delicious meal into a pang of regret that you ate too much. The harsh burning in your chest and icky gush of saliva in your mouth can also rob you of a restful night's sleep.

But heartburn isn't merely a painful annoyance; in rare cases it can be an early signpost on the road to esophageal cancer.

Your esophagus is the muscular tunnel that carries food from your mouth down to your stomach. At the bottom of the esophagus, between it and your stomach, a valve (called a *sphincter,* but "valve" sounds nicer) keeps stomach contents in the stomach. Since your stomach is designed to handle the acid and other harsh elements that it contains, and your esophagus isn't, this valve is a mighty handy device.

However, sometimes the valve doesn't stay closed as tightly as it should, and it allows stomach fluids to rise into the esophagus. You might notice it as heartburn. Doctors call this wayward activity "reflux," and when it happens chronically it's called gastroesophageal reflux disease, or GERD for short.

Your esophagus might respond to this assault by changing cells in its lining to cells that look more like those found in the intestine. This alteration is called "Barrett's esophagus," and you want to avoid it.

Barrett's esophagus seems to set the stage for a type of cancer called esophageal adenocarcinoma. According to the National Institutes of Health, the risk of developing adenocarcinoma is 30 to 125 times greater in people with Barrett's esophagus than in those without it.

Don't Let Barrett's Sneak Up on You

While aspirin might be an interesting idea in preventing esophageal cancer, your doctor can take a number of steps that are known to protect you from complications of reflux.

Start by knowing the signs of reflux: You may feel heartburn and hoarseness in the morning. You may also have difficulty swallowing and feel like food gets stuck in your throat while you're eating. Reflux disease, or GERD, can also cause dry mouth and bad breath, according to the National Institutes of Health.

Smoking and alcohol use may make you more likely to develop GERD, and so can being overweight.

Your doctor may suggest or prescribe a number of medications to treat the problem, including over-the-counter antacids; drugs called "H2 blockers," like Tagamet, Pepcid, or Zantac; or "proton pump inhibitors" such as Prilosec or Nexium.

A more advanced step to treat the problem is surgery to strengthen the sphincter that separates the bottom of the esophagus from the stomach.

A doctor can monitor how much acid you have rising into your esophagus and how much damage it's caused through a number of methods, including inspecting the area with a tiny camera that goes down through your mouth.

Although it's an uncommon disease, the number of people getting this cancer in the esophagus and where it meets the stomach is on the rise in America. The rates have tripled in the past thirty years, according to Douglas Corley, M.D., Ph.D., M.P.H., an assistant clinical professor of medicine at the University of California in San Francisco, who studies GERD and esophageal cancer.

This type of cancer is quite deadly. It's often not detected until it's in an advanced stage, at which point people have only about a 14 percent chance of surviving another five years.

"And it's not showing any sign of going down, just continued straight up," he says. Reflux disease is associated with being overweight (the added pressure in the abdomen pushes stomach contents upward), and the epidemic numbers of overweight people in the country may be playing a role in the growing incidence of the disease.

Early evidence, however, points to aspirin as a possible method of reducing the likelihood of developing this form of cancer.

In 2003, Dr. Corley published a study with colleagues examining the possible role of aspirin in minimizing the disease's development.

His meta-analysis—or paper summarizing the results of other studies—found that aspirin use was associated with a 50 percent reduction in the risk of esophageal carcinomas. More aspirin use was associated with greater protection.

Previous research discovered a link between greater amounts of the COX-2 enzyme and the development of Barrett's esophagus and its progression to cancer. The enzyme could help the cancer along by inhibiting apoptosis—the cells' command to die at a specific time—or by helping it develop blood vessels to feed it nutrients, according to the current scientific reasoning, Dr. Corley says.

Aspirin may help by limiting the activity of the COX-2 enzyme, thus preventing its cancer-aiding potential. It also might decrease the inflammation that comes from the stomach contents making contact with the throat, and this anti-inflammatory action could be totally aside from COX-2 inhibition.

Thus, according to Dr. Corley, the aspirin might protect you by preventing Barrett's esophagus in the first place, or by keeping it from turning into cancer. However, more research—particularly randomized controlled trials—is needed to offer more support of these findings.

Another study, published in 2004, examined whether aspirin use would be a cost-effective way to prevent esophageal adenocarcinoma if, in fact, aspirin really does offer a 50 percent reduction in the risk of the disease.

The study, by Chin Hur, M.D., M.P.H., an instructor of medicine at Harvard Medical School, and colleagues, concluded with the suggestion that in the average patient with Barrett's esophagus, "aspirin use may be a reasonable recommendation," provided that future studies show that it gives at least a 50 percent protection against the cancer. If the person also has risk factors for heart disease, aspirin may be an "obvious recommendation."

It's this cost-effectiveness that makes aspirin particularly attractive as a tool against esophageal cancer—perhaps even more so than in colorectal cancer, Dr. Corley says. As far as the colon goes, doing screenings to find and remove polyps before they turn dangerous is effective, thus it preserves people's quality of life and saves money by preventing cancer. Taking aspirin might not prove to be any more cost-effective for the public than cancer screenings, when you figure in the cost of treating the complications from aspirin in some people.

However, the same safety net doesn't exist for esophageal cancer. A doctor can check the esophagus for cancer, but can't easily remove the esophagus if a cancer does arise, Dr. Corley points out. Thus using aspirin to bring down a person's risk for the disease might make more sense in this instance, both from a cost perspective and by adding quality years to people's lives.

STOMACH CANCER

Cancer of the stomach—also known as gastric cancer—is actually becoming more rare in the United States; death rates from the disease dropped markedly between 1930 and 2000, according to the American Cancer Society.

In 1930, it was the most common cause of cancer death in the United States. It's now the fourteenth most common cancer, and the eighth leading cause of cancer death in the country. It's a much larger problem in some other countries such as Japan and some former Soviet countries.

A common household appliance has played a major role in the reduction in stomach cancer in America. Want to guess what it is?

It's not the television.

It's not the microwave, but that's getting closer.

It's the refrigerator. Eating lots of pickled, salted, and smoked foods raises your risk of stomach cancer. Once people started storing their food in refrigerators, they didn't have to eat so many preserved items.

Another factor that puts you at higher risk of the disease is the *H. pylori* bacterium. This germ is able to live in the harsh environment of your stomach, where it burrows into the organ's mucous lining. The bacteria and the acid in your stomach cause irritated spots in the lining. If that sounds like an ulcer, you're right—most peptic ulcers are thought to be caused by *H. pylori*.

H. pylori may also make you several times more likely to have stomach cancer. The chronic inflammation in the stomach—true to what we've already learned in this chapter—can cause unusual cell growth that progresses to cancer.

Though the chance of developing the disease has fallen in America, your odds of surviving long if you do get stomach cancer are poor: You have about a 20 percent chance of living with it for five years.

More than 90 percent of stomach cancers are adenocarcinomas, which begin on the epithelial cells lining your stomach. They can grow into and through the wall of your stomach, where they can spread to other organs or get into the lymph system.

Aspirin and other NSAIDs have been linked with a lower risk of developing stomach cancer.

In a 2003 report in the *Journal of the National Cancer Institute,* a team of researchers in Beijing and Hong Kong reviewed a group of nine studies that explored the relationship between stomach cancer and the drugs.

When they pooled the results of these studies together, they found that aspirin use was associated with a 27 percent smaller risk of having stomach cancer. Plus, people who used NSAIDs regularly had a lower risk than those who took them less often.

According to the authors, the COX-2 enzyme may play a role in stomach cancer by encouraging more cell division, discouraging cell death, and increasing blood vessel growth to tumors.

However, the study had a number of limitations—or factors that may have led the researchers to incorrect conclusions. But more research into aspirin's effects on reducing stomach cancer may prove to be particularly helpful in parts of the world where the people are at high risk of the disease.

OTHER STRATEGIES

You don't have to wait to reduce your risk of the cancers in this chapter until the experts give you the go-ahead to use aspirin. Plenty of other steps can help, too, according to the American Cancer Society:

Colorectal Cancer

- Be screened for polyps and cancer following the schedules provided on page 94.
- Exercise for at least thirty minutes at least five days a week.
- Eat a diet that's rich in whole grains and fruits and vegetables, and low in fat.
- Take a daily multivitamin containing folic acid, and increase your calcium and vitamin D intake with supplements or low-fat dairy foods.

    All might reduce your risk.

Stomach Cancer

- Avoid making smoked and pickled foods and salted meat and fish a major part of your diet.
- Consider being tested for the *H. pylori* germ and getting treated if you have it.
- Eat a diet high in fruits, vegetables, and whole grains.
- Avoid smoking, and if you must drink, keep it in moderation.

Esophageal Cancer

- Avoid smoking and drinking alcohol.
- Eat a diet heavy in fruits and vegetables.
- Maintain a healthy body weight.
- If you have Barrett's esophagus, have your doctor test you regularly to observe whether abnormal cells are progressing toward cancer.

8

Breast Cancer

A common refrain among women who've just returned from getting a mammogram is that *some man* surely invented this method of detecting breast cancer.

This process involves X-raying the breast while it's pressed between two plates to hold it in place, produce a sharper image, and reduce the amount of radiation needed for the picture. It can be a real eye-opener. A survey of 1,800 California women who'd recently undergone a mammogram found that slightly more than half had experienced "moderate to extreme discomfort."

The next time you leave a breast-cancer checkup thinking bad things about "the guy" who invented the uncomfortable process, you can direct your thoughts to Raul Leborgne, a Uruguayan physician who deserves at least some of the credit. Back in 1949, he promoted the practice of compressing the breasts to better detect possible signs of cancer inside them.

Until 1966, mammograms were done with regular X-ray equipment. Then a special device just for X-raying breasts was devised. In the early 1980s, a motorized device for compressing the breasts was developed, immortalizing Dr. Leborgne's legacy. Though the mammogram may not be fun, it saves a lot of women pain and heartache later. The process is the best way to find cancer at the earliest stages, before it has spread into surrounding tissues, and when it's almost always successfully treated.

If you take aspirin regularly, the next time you breathe a sigh of relief that your mammogram found you cancer-free, you might *also* want to think a good thought about the guy who discovered aspirin. (That would be Felix Hoffmann, if you skipped chapter 1.)

Researchers are finding that women who take aspirin may be less likely to develop breast cancer. Given that breast cancer is so common, this possibility of aspirin is attracting a lot of attention.

After skin cancer, breast cancer is the type most commonly found in women. It struck roughly 216,000 women in 2004. And it's the second most frequent cause of cancer death in women, after lung cancer. The disease killed about 41,000 women in 2004.

Breast cancer isn't restricted solely to women; a small number of cases are found in men. But since women's burden of this disease is about 100 times larger (470 men died of breast cancer in 2004), we'll be using the pronouns "she" and "her" in this chapter when referring to people with breast cancer.

Before looking into how aspirin might make women less likely to get breast cancer, let's look at how the disease develops.

Your Breasts: What's Inside Them in Health and Sickness

A cross-section of the breast, when viewed from the side, reveals structures that look like tree roots burrowing into the breast from the nipple. These "roots" are hollow ducts that lead from the nipple to milk-producing glands called "lobules."

Each nipple is perforated with five to ten openings, each of which leads to a system of ducts, which branches out to smaller and smaller ducts, which lead to the lobules. A woman may have a million lobules in each breast.

Breasts also contain fat, blood vessels, connective tissue, and vessels that carry lymph—a fluid containing immune cells and wastes from tissues—out to lymph nodes, mostly located in the underarms and around the collarbones. The lymph nodes filter out bacteria and cancer cells and create immune-system cells to fight infections.

About 80 percent of breast cancers develop in the ducts leading from the lobules to the nipple, and about 20 percent develop in the lobules.

The Aspirin Vocabulary

- *Aromatase.* An enzyme that helps in the production of estrogen, which is a particularly important process in how postmenopausal women get the hormone.
- *Carcinoma in situ.* This is an early stage of cancer, when it's still confined to where it began. Ductal carcinoma in situ is almost always curable. Lobular carcinoma isn't a true cancer, but some experts consider it to be a cancer that hasn't spread.
- *Duct.* The tube leading from a lobule to the nipple, through which milk travels. The most common kind of breast cancer starts here.
- *Estrogen.* A hormone that's mainly made by the ovaries, which plays a role in the menstrual cycle and monthly breast changes. It can also play a role in breast cancer.
- *Estrogen receptor.* A protein found in some breast cells, and breast cancer cells, where estrogen can attach and cause the cells to divide.
- *Lobule.* Tiny sac-like gland that produces milk. These can be the site of cancer.
- *Progesterone.* Another hormone made by the ovaries. It, too, may play a role in breast cancer.

Breast cancer is classified two different ways, depending on whether it's sitting in one place or spreading out, according to the American Cancer Society:

- *Carcinoma in situ.* This is an early stage at which abnormal cells are found in a duct (thus called ductal carcinoma in situ) or lobule (lobular carcinoma in situ), but haven't spread beyond the duct or lobe into other tissues. The best way to find the ductal form is with a mammogram, and nearly all women can be cured at this stage, according to the ACS. The lobular form isn't actually considered a true cancer, but it can turn into one.
- *Invasive cancer.* A cancer in a duct or lobule grows out into surrounding tissue, where it can spread to other parts of the body. Invasive ductal carcinoma represents about 80 percent of invasive breast cancer.

Cancerous cells can spread to distant parts of the body after they get into the bloodstream or the lymphatic system. Cancer is caused by cells that don't grow in an orderly fashion like they're supposed to—they instead grow and divide excessively and refuse to die on time. These growths, or tumors, can develop blood vessels that feed them, depriving healthy tissue of nutrients. For more on how cancers begin and grow in general, see page 98.

It's worth remembering here that not all lumps in the breast are cancerous. Women may also detect fluid-filled cysts, lumpy scar tissue, or other noncancerous knots in their breasts.

A woman's hormones may play a role in breast cancer development. Being exposed to estrogen and progesterone—hormones produced by the ovaries—can increase a woman's risk of breast cancer. Women who began puberty early, never had children, or entered menopause late—all of which increase their exposure to these hormones—have a higher risk of the disease.

To see how this works (don't worry, we're only covering it because aspirin will figure in later), we'll look at estrogen. Molecules of estrogen in a woman's body have effects on a number of her organs, particularly her uterus and breasts.

Cells in the tissues in these organs have "estrogen receptors." You can think of these as little locks in the cells, and the only keys that will fit into them are estrogen molecules, or something similar to them. When an estrogen molecule gets into one of these cells and fits into an estrogen receptor, it can spark the DNA inside the cell to start making the cell perform a particular activity.

During each menstrual cycle, estrogen makes cells in the milk glands in the breasts proliferate—or reproduce by dividing—to get the breasts ready to produce milk in case the woman gets pregnant. If she doesn't get pregnant that month, her estrogen drops and those extra cells die off.

Should cells in this woman's breasts develop mutations in their DNA that send them on the path toward becoming cancerous, the estrogen will increase the number of these odd cells that have the potential to become cancer.

Women with receptor-positive tumors tend to have a better chance for effective treatment than those whose tumors don't have the receptors.

Not all breast-cancer tumors contain hormone receptors. When doctors remove a tumor, they can now check whether it has the receptors or not. Tumors that have the estrogen or progesterone receptors are called ER or PR positive. A tumor with both is called ER/PR positive.

A type of drug called SERM—for selective estrogen receptor modulator—can reduce the risk of breast cancer in women who've had the disease or are at higher risk for it. One well-known SERM is tamoxifen (Nolvadex). It fits into estrogen receptors in cells and keeps estrogen from being able to slide in. In the breasts, this keeps those cells from proliferating when they come into contact with estrogen.

Some drugs target these receptors to fight cancer, but aspirin interferes with estrogen in a different way. Here's how it can help.

ASPIRIN: A POSSIBLE MONKEY WRENCH IN CANCER'S PLANS

As in the cancers discussed in the previous chapter, aspirin may work against breast tumors by shutting down the COX-2 enzyme in the body. The COX enzyme—which comes in at least two forms—helps you create chemicals called prostaglandins, which work like hormones. These play both beneficial and harmful roles in your body.

COX-2 may help breast cancer develop by contributing to cell mutations, encouraging cell division, promoting tumor growth, suppressing the immune system, and helping cancer cells spread to other locations.

COX-1 is seen as a protector, always around as part of a normal system. COX-2 generally pops up when things are out of whack, like during inflammation and cancer. So it's interesting that research has found COX-2 in breast tumors, but not in normal breast tissue. And the more COX-2 a tumor has, the denser the cancer cells in the tumor are.

"Why COX-2 gets turned on and stuck in the on position in cancer cells is a major question that still remains to be answered. The molecular studies are quite convincing that if you turn on COX-2, you stimulate a variety of elements of carcinogenesis big-time. You stimulate angiogenesis (blood-vessel growth to feed cancer cells), and you stimulate a lack of apoptosis, which means the cells don't die like they're supposed to. You also stimulate metastasis, or invasion into other tissues," says Randall Harris, M.D., Ph.D., a professor of epidemiology and cancer expert at Ohio State University in Columbus. "It certainly is promoting carcinogenesis in a variety of ways, and the ultimate fact is that COX-2 being turned on may elevate the risk of mutations," he says.

Aspirin permanently alters the COX enzyme, making it unable to assist in producing prostaglandins. Therefore, it reduces your prostaglandin levels.

Another way aspirin might help in fighting breast cancer is by reducing the amount of estrogen in the body. Premenopausal women get most of their estrogen directly from their ovaries. But their hormonal production stops at menopause.

After that, some estrogen still remains present in your body, since tissues in your body convert a chemical called androstenedione made by your adrenal glands into estrogen. However, the enzyme called *aromatase* is required in the process of making estrogen this way. The presence of a prostaglandin (more specifically, prostaglandin E2, if you really enjoy the details) increases aromatase. Thus, a breast tumor with a lot of COX-2 can help generate more estrogen, thus multiplying its cells.

One study that looked at twenty-three breast tumors found that COX-2 and the presence of aromatase had a "significant positive correlation," which means that as the COX-2 went up, so did the aromatase.

So aspirin may help reduce your risk of breast cancer by inhibiting the COX enzyme, thus reducing prostaglandins, thus reducing the aromatase, thus reducing estrogen, which may reduce the multiplication of cancer cells in receptor-positive tumors.

Pretty heady stuff for such a common drug.

"If you turn on COX-2 in the ductal epithelium (the thin lining of the ducts) of the mammary gland, you've got a direct route to estrogen creation locally . . . and you have an abundance of estrogen there that shouldn't really be there," Dr. Harris says. "Estrogen is a powerful, powerful mitogen, or cell-division factor. It's the most powerful cell-division factor that we know of!"

The idea of such a familiar, easy-to-obtain drug interfering with cancer in so many ways sounds great . . . but how well does it work in the real world?

WHAT THE STUDIES ARE SHOWING

From Iowa to Long Island to England, evidence is growing that women who take aspirin and other nonsteroidal anti-inflammatory drugs (NSAIDs) have less breast cancer.

In 2002, a team of researchers from the University of Minnesota published a study in which they'd pored over data on nearly 30,000 Iowan women who'd gone through menopause.

Women who reported on a questionnaire that they were currently using two to five aspirin weekly turned out to be 20 percent less likely to develop breast cancer over the next six years. The more aspirin the women took, the lower their risk of breast cancer appeared to be:

Those who took six or more aspirin a week had almost 30 percent less risk. The researchers found no association between other kinds of NSAIDs—like Advil and Motrin—and risk of breast cancer.

Another long-running study—the Women's Health Initiative (WHI)—also turned its attention to the possible effects of aspirin and other NSAIDs on women's breast cancer risk. The WHI was launched in 1991 by the National Institutes of Health, and it involved an "observational study" to examine a number of possible risk factors that could play a role in heart disease, cancer, and fractures in women.

Led by Dr. Harris, researchers analyzing data from nearly 81,000 postmenopausal women enrolled in the WHI published a study on aspirin and breast cancer in 2003. They found that using NSAIDs at a rate of two or more tablets a week for five to nine years was associated with a 21 percent reduction in the risk of breast cancer. Using them for ten or more years gave a 28 percent reduction.

However, in this study, long-term use of ibuprofen gave a greater reduction in risk than aspirin (49 percent less risk versus 21 percent).

Another study, published in 2004, looked at women ages thirty to seventy-nine from England. Researchers pored through a vast, extensive computer database of medical records that the government maintains and came up with a group of more than 730,000 women treated during a six-year period to analyze.

Roughly 3,700 women were diagnosed with breast cancer in this time period. The authors then proceeded to do a case-control study using these women. In this type of study, researchers take a group of people with a particular condition and compare them to a group of people with similar characteristics such as age and gender *without* the disease. The researchers try to see if the people with and without the disease did something different or were exposed to something different that could have made them more or less likely to develop the disease.

So the researchers compared the 3,700 women who'd had breast cancer to 20,000 who hadn't. They found that women who took aspirin for a year or longer were 23 percent less likely to have breast cancer. The authors, however, didn't find any association between non-aspirin NSAIDs and a reduced risk of breast cancer.

Yet another study from 2004, published in the *Journal of the Amer-*

ican Medical Association, added more detail on who might stand to benefit the most from aspirin to prevent breast cancer. (It also provides the reason why we talked about hormone receptor-positive tumors earlier.)

Conducted by Mary Beth Terry, Ph.D., an assistant professor of public health at Columbia University in New York, this case-control study compared 1,442 women from Long Island who'd had breast cancer with 1,420 controls, who hadn't had the disease. Three hundred and one women who'd had breast cancer had taken aspirin at least once a week for six months or more. Three hundred forty-five women who *hadn't* had breast cancer had taken it for this long.

By running this finding through their statistical models, the researchers concluded that taking aspirin weekly for at least six months was associated with a 20 percent smaller risk of breast cancer. The women who took at least seven aspirin tablets weekly had nearly a 30 percent smaller risk of breast cancer. They also looked at the association of ibuprofen with breast cancer, which showed a weaker effect.

The researchers also collected information from pathology reports written on the women who'd had breast cancer, to find out whether their tumors had hormone receptors. This allowed them to break the findings down to see if the aspirin effect applied equally to all the women, whether or not their tumors were positive for hormone receptors.

It didn't. The reduction in risk was only seen in women with hormone-receptor-positive tumors. This lends support to the idea that aspirin can help prevent breast cancer by reducing the amount of estrogen in a woman's body that could contribute to the production of cancerous cells.

Though roughly eighteen studies have been conducted on aspirin and breast cancer, and all are consistent in suggesting a decrease in risk of about 30 to 40 percent from aspirin, this study attracted a lot of attention from the media, Dr. Terry says.

"People are always looking for that magic pill, and in breast cancer, there aren't a lot of risk factors that are modifiable—a lot depend on reproductive factors," she says. In other words, you can't change when you begin puberty or menopause, and you're unlikely to have babies just to lower your breast cancer risk.

The drug tamoxifen has been shown to lower your risk more than aspirin might, but it also has more side effects, Dr. Terry says, such as slightly raising your risk of some uterine cancers, as well as possibly raising your risk of blood clots, which could cause a stroke.

But the time still hasn't arrived for experts to advise women to take aspirin for breast cancer prevention purposes, she says.

Why not? Why can't doctors just recommend aspirin, a common, familiar drug, to prevent such a horrible disease, since so many studies have shown possible protection? Because, she explains, epidemiological studies that observe people's behaviors and make calculations from them can be "crude" instruments for supporting recommendations.

For example, consider the case of hormone replacement therapy. The bulk of studies that supported the use of estrogen and progestin in menopausal women to control their hot flashes, prevent osteoporosis, and keep a handle on other menopause-related conditions were based on epidemiological data, Dr. Terry says.

Then in 2002 came a bombshell that frightened women nationwide. A major study sponsored by the National Institutes of Health, looking at the use of these hormones to prevent heart disease and fractures, was halted early. The study, involving more than 16,000 women who hadn't undergone hysterectomies, found that not only did the hormones not protect the women's hearts—they increased their risk of breast cancer, to boot.

The risks exceeded the benefits, in other words. And because this was a randomized controlled study, the researchers were able to control whether the women actually took the drug, as opposed to observational studies, where participants' inaccurate recall of what drugs they took and for how long can lead to shaky conclusions. The evidence was now solid that this therapy, which had been thought to be protective, wasn't.

The medical establishment isn't eager to repeat this experience, and recommendations for aspirin in breast cancer are going to have to wait for additional lines of evidence from both laboratory and epidemiological research.

So for now, popping aspirin to prevent breast cancer remains an intriguing possibility. But if you have reason to take aspirin for other valid uses, such as heart protection, you may enjoy some peace of mind that the drug may also be protecting your breast health, too.

Until you get the go-ahead from your doctor to use aspirin specifically for breast cancer protection, reduce your risk with the ideas below.

OTHER STRATEGIES

If you'd like to reduce your risk of breast cancer, aspirin isn't the only option that could help. Consider the following steps, recommended by the American Cancer Society.

- Talk to your doctor if you're at higher risk of cancer about whether you might benefit from the drug tamoxifen (Nolvadex) to reduce your risk. Some risk factors include being middle-aged or older; having a personal history or family history of breast cancer; having a certain genetic mutation; or beginning menstruation earlier than twelve; having no children or having your first late in life; or going through menopause after age fifty-five.
- If you have a particularly high risk of developing breast cancer, you may find the idea of preventive mastectomy, or breast removal, acceptable in lowering your risk of the disease.

9

Other Cancers

Though researchers haven't discovered as much evidence linking aspirin use to the prevention of the diseases in this chapter as they've found for colorectal and breast cancer, they have found some interesting signs that the drug could be helpful.

Considering that roughly 250,000 people died of the cancers in this chapter in 2004—and that some of these ailments have few, if any, symptoms in their early stages, yet are terrifyingly deadly when they're advanced—aspirin's potential in reducing your risk of these diseases is certainly interesting.

"Across the board, I think you'd have to say that aspirin and other NSAIDs have tremendous potential in reducing the risk of a variety of malignancies," says Randall Harris, M.D., Ph.D., an Ohio State University professor who has directed a number of studies looking at aspirin in cancer prevention, including early studies on lung cancer and prostate cancer prevention.

"It's not just breast cancer, it's not just colorectal cancer, it's not just esophageal cancer. (NSAIDs) have an effect across a variety of malignancies—oral cavity malignancies, ovarian cancer, cervical cancer, malignant melanoma. You name it and there probably is a study out there showing a protective effective of either aspirin or some of the other selective COX-2 blockers in either human beings or animals or cell lines," he says.

Here's a look at some of the types of cancer for which scientists have studied the use of aspirin in recent years for prevention.

LEUKEMIA

Leukemia is cancer of cells in the bone marrow that are in charge of creating different kinds of blood cells. The cancer can spread through the bloodstream and lymphatic system to affect other organs, including the liver and brain. The disease comes in several different forms, depending on which type of cell in the bone marrow is not dividing on a normal schedule, and whether cells are undeveloped or partially developed when they divide.

Leukemia killed roughly 23,300 Americans in 2004. Not much is known about what causes the disease.

In 2003 a team of researchers from the University of Minnesota looked into whether aspirin may help protect adults from the disease, having determined that few studies had investigated the possible connections between the drug and leukemia.

More than 28,000 women filled out a questionnaire in 1992 that asked, among other things, about their use of aspirin and other non-steroidal anti-inflammatory drugs. The researchers then noted how many of the women developed leukemia between 1993 and 2000. Eighty-one came down with the disease.

The women who took aspirin at least twice a week had 55 percent less risk of leukemia than women who took none.

However, since the study relied on women to remember their history of aspirin use, the results may have been affected if subjects didn't remember properly. Plus, since the study only looked at women between the ages of fifty-five and sixty-nine, the results might not apply to other types of people.

More and larger studies will be needed to look into what role, if any, aspirin might play in this disease.

LUNG CANCER

Since 1987, more women have died annually from lung cancer than breast cancer, which had been the largest cause of cancer death for women for the previous forty years, according to the American Cancer Society.

This is the kind of cancer that kills more people each year than any other. More than one-quarter of cancer deaths in 2004 were due to lung cancer, claiming about 160,000 people, according to ACS figures.

The biggest risk factor in lung cancer, not surprisingly, is smoking. Even breathing secondhand smoke can raise the risk in people who don't practice the habit themselves.

Some laboratory evidence suggests that aspirin could be helpful in preventing lung cancer; scientists have learned, for example, that aspirin can limit the formation of lung tumors in animals. Also, prostaglandin levels—which aspirin reduces—have been found to be higher in lung tumors than in healthy surrounding tissue.

> The five-year survival rate for lung cancer, from early to advanced combined, is only about 15 percent. If doctors catch the cancer when it's still in its original spot and hasn't spread, the survival rate is nearly 50 percent—but they're not frequently diagnosed at this early stage.

Studies of large groups of people, assessing their use of aspirin and their rates of lung cancer, have come up with conflicting results. Some have shown that the drug may reduce the risk of the disease and some haven't. However, some outside factors may have affected these studies' ability to estimate the true relationship—such as subjects' smoking habits, or a small number of cancers that arise during the study period, which provides a smaller amount of data to examine.

One 2002 study, however, found some positive news by looking at more than 14,000 New York women enrolled in a long-term project to investigate risk factors of cancer. The women answered questionnaires about their use of aspirin. The researchers then compared data from the eighty-one women who developed lung cancer during the study period with 808 women of similar age and menopausal status who remained free of lung cancer during the study period.

They found that taking aspirin three or more times a week for at least six months was associated with a lower risk of cancer. The association was even stronger for the risk of a type of lung cancer called the non-small cell type, which is the most common kind; women taking aspirin regularly had a 60 percent lower risk.

Another case-control study, this one from a 2003 issue of the journal *Cancer*, compared 1,038 patients with lung cancer with 1,002 people without the disease, and also looked at their use of aspirin and other NSAIDs.

Researchers found that people who had smoked at some point in their lives—and had taken aspirin at least three times a week for at least a year—had a 32 percent smaller chance of having lung cancer.

The authors surmise that smoking could trigger COX-2 production, which is how aspirin could play some type of protective role.

"The ultimate answer whether aspirin is beneficial against cancer will come from randomized clinical trials," says Alan A. Arslan, M.D., of the New York University School of Medicine, who was the lead researcher on the 2002 study of New York women. These are studies in which the researchers give aspirin or placebo to the subjects, then estimate the effectiveness of aspirin in prevention of cancer compared to placebo.

> However, the authors of a study that didn't find any association between aspirin and lung cancer said that a better way to avoid lung cancer than taking aspirin is to simply not start smoking, or quit the habit if you already smoke.

"There are ongoing clinical trials right now on aspirin and some other cancers that are trying to answer this question," he says.

LYMPHOMA

This cancer affects organs of the immune system, such as the lymph nodes and spleen. It involves abnormal growth of lymphocytes, which are white blood cells that help recognize and destroy invading cells in your body. These circulate in your bloodstream and lymphatic system, including your lymph nodes, which are scattered throughout your body but are found in clusters in your armpits and groin.

This disease comes in two types: Hodgkin's lymphoma and non-Hodgkin's lymphoma. Non-Hodgkin's is far more common and claims far more lives. In 2004, roughly 1,320 people died of Hodgkin's, and 19,410 died of non-Hodgkin's.

A 2004 case-control study in the *Journal of the National Cancer Institute* looked for the first time—as far as the authors could surmise—at whether there's any link between NSAID use and Hodgkin's disease.

According to the authors, the COX enzyme—which is required to create prostaglandins in your body, which may have harmful effects—is found in higher amounts in cancerous cells in Hodgkin's disease. Elevated prostaglandin levels are also found in higher levels in Hodgkin's tumors. Aspirin disables the COX enzyme from forming prostaglandins.

Aspirin also inhibits a protein called a *transcription factor* that's involved in the copying of genetic material during cell division. This transcription factor is almost always found in an activated form in Hodgkin's cells, and blocking this turned-on transcription factor causes spontaneous cell death of Hodgkin's cells.

The researchers surveyed 565 people in Boston and Connecticut with Hodgkin's (these were the cases), and 679 people who didn't have the disease, but were similar in age, gender, and state of residence (these were the controls). They asked the subjects about their use of aspirin and other NSAIDs over the previous five years.

The researchers found that taking at least two aspirins a week on average over the previous five years was associated with a 40 percent less risk of the disease compared to taking less than two aspirins weekly. The more aspirin people took, the lower the risk. The use of other NSAIDs had no effect on the risk of the disease.

"The finding that regular aspirin use is associated with a decreased risk of Hodgkin's lymphoma is intriguing," the authors note. If indeed aspirin does help protect against Hodgkin's lymphoma, it could help give researchers more ideas about what causes the condition, and possibly how to prevent it.

OVARIAN CANCER

This type of cancer is quiet but deadly. The early symptoms of cancer are vague and are the kinds of complaints often caused by minor ailments, such as back pain, gas, and bloating.

It's also virtually impossible for a doctor to feel an ovarian tumor in the early stages while giving a woman a pelvic exam. Other screening methods aren't particularly helpful in detecting it, either. As a result, nearly 70 percent of women with the most common kind of ovarian cancer, which starts in the epithelial lining covering the ovaries, don't find out they have the disease until it's advanced. The five-year survival rate once the cancer has spread in the upper abdomen or beyond is only 20 percent or less.

As a result, if experts want to reduce ovarian-cancer deaths, preventing it is a smart approach, and aspirin is a possible candidate to do the job.

Following up on evidence that indicates ovarian cancer might be connected to inflammation, researchers from New York published a case-control study in 2001 looking for links between aspirin and ovarian-cancer protection.

They used data from a long-running prospective study of New York women and found sixty-eight who'd developed epithelial ovarian cancer. They then assembled a group of 680 women from the study who didn't have ovarian cancer, but were similar in terms of age and whether they'd gone through menopause. They also reviewed their history of aspirin usage.

Women who reported taking aspirin at least three times a week for at least six months were 40 percent less likely to develop epithelial ovarian cancer. However, according to the results it's statistically possible that the observed relationship actually was due to chance.

Aspirin's preventive effects are difficult to study in ovarian cancer, says Dr. Arslan, who was the lead researcher. Ovarian cancer is relatively uncommon, making it more difficult to study prospectively. Plus, since aspirin is so easily available and commonly consumed, it's hard for subjects to remember how long they took it and at what dose.

However, it makes sense that it could work in this type of ovarian cancer, since "the similar preventive mechanism may be applicable to many epithelial cancers," such as those in the colon, he says, where aspirin has shown stronger evidence of cancer prevention. Experts think inflammation may play a role in epithelial ovarian cancer.

According to Dr. Arslan, prostaglandins are involved in local inflammation and they can stimulate epithelial cells to divide and also interfere with the immune system's ability to shut down cancerous cells. Aspirin could play a beneficial role in ovarian cancer by inhibiting COX enzymes and limiting the production of prostaglandins. It also may help through non-COX-related mechanisms. Since aspirin has been shown to trigger normal cell death in epithelial cells, it could be helpful by inducing the death of rogue cells that are involved in ovarian cancer.

PROSTATE CANCER

According to the American Cancer Society, prostate cancer is the most common form of cancer in men in America, other than skin cancer. It accounts for roughly one-third of all male cancer diagnoses each year, and is the second-leading cause of cancer death in men, after lung cancer. In 2004, nearly 30,000 American men died of it.

The disease is far more common in older men—it seldom strikes under the age of forty—and a man's risk of getting the disease rises as he ages.

The COX-2 enzyme has been found to be overproduced in cancerous prostate tissue compared to healthy tissue. It could help cancer develop and progress by decreasing normal cell death and stimulating cell growth.

In 2004, a pair of Spanish researchers published a case-control study, using data on British men, to show an association between aspirin and a lower risk of prostate cancer. Poring through a vast database of medical records on more than two million patients, they identified 2,183 cases of prostate cancer. They used 10,000 men of similar ages who didn't have prostate cancer as controls, then looked at records of aspirin prescriptions for the men (according to the authors, the subjects' unknown over-the-counter aspirin use wouldn't affect the findings).

The results showed that using aspirin was associated with a 30 percent reduction in risk of prostate cancer.

Another study, also from 2004, analyzed twelve studies that looked at the relationship between NSAIDs and prostate cancer and found that overall the use of aspirin was associated with a 10 percent lower risk of prostate cancer. However, the authors note, the studies didn't show consistent results—some of them showed no association between aspirin and cancer risk.

Section V

Fertility

Thus far we've talked about how aspirin can help make you healthier. In the following section, however, you'll learn how aspirin might possibly help someone else: Your unborn child, if you're pregnant.

Researchers around the world are investigating whether aspirin might help prevent a relatively common pregnancy complication, and whether the drug can help make an expensive fertility treatment more likely to work. And they're finding evidence pointing out that it's useful in both cases.

10

Preeclampsia and
In Vitro Fertilization

When aspirin made its debut in America at the turn of the twentieth century, the nation was beginning a major change in how it brought its babies into the world.

In 1900, fewer than 5 percent of babies were born in hospitals in the United States. Midwives—who varied widely in their training, experience, and literacy—had traditionally attended births in the home over the course of the nation's history. At the turn of the century, they still attended about half of all births, more frequently when the family was poor.

Physicians coming out of medical school in the early 1900s tended to be poorly trained to handle births, and preventable infections were common among mothers who gave birth in hospitals, due to doctors who didn't wash their hands properly between patients.

However, the practice of medicine became standardized, organized, specialized, and powerful in the early part of the century. Doctors began using anesthetics, forceps, and other medicines and tools to manage some of the pain and complications of childbirth, and they began convincing society that the process should be handled as a medical issue.

Now, of course, childbirth is typically a high-tech affair. Pregnant women track their babies' growth and development with ultrasound pictures, which are now available in detailed 3-D movies. Doctors can start contractions with medications. During childbirth, women are hooked up to fetal heart monitors and offered their choice of a range of anesthesia options to prevent pain. In the event of complications, doctors have a host of treatments to keep the mother healthy, and intensive-care options to keep the baby stable. In addition, nearly a quarter of babies in the United States are surgically delivered by cesarean section.

But even though childbirth has changed radically in the last one hundred years or so, involving technology that would have been unimaginable a few generations ago, aspirin can still play a role in treating and preventing reproductive problems.

Though you shouldn't use aspirin if you're pregnant without getting your doctor's approval, the drug has been found useful in preventing a serious condition called preeclampsia; it may give couples more success from in vitro fertilization; and it's been associated with a lower risk of low birth weight.

USING ASPIRIN TO CLAMP DOWN ON PREECLAMPSIA

Preeclampsia (pronounced pre-eh-*klamp*-see-eh) is a potentially serious condition that can threaten the health—and life—of a pregnant woman and her baby. It affects roughly 6 percent of all pregnancies. Women at higher risk of the condition include first-time mothers, African Americans, women pregnant with more than one baby, and those with high blood pressure going into the pregnancy.

Though in its mild forms it may cause no symptoms, women with preeclampsia may notice blurred vision, headaches, sudden weight gain (like a pound a day), and swelling of the hands and feet. However, swollen feet are also common in pregnant women without the condition.

The Aspirin Vocabulary

- *Eclampsia.* A complication of preeclampsia, this condition is marked by seizures. It can cause permanent damage to vital organs and can be fatal to the mother and baby.
- *Preeclampsia.* A serious condition found during pregnancy that's marked by high blood pressure and protein in the urine caused by kidney malfunction. The only way to cure it is to deliver the baby.
- *Prostacyclin.* A chemical made by the lining of blood vessels from prostaglandin that discourages clotting. It normally counterbalances the effects of thromboxane.
- *Thromboxane.* A chemical made from platelets in the blood from prostaglandin that promotes platelet clumping, clotting, and blood-vessel tightening.

Two signs a doctor looks for to diagnose preeclampsia are high blood pressure and protein in the urine. That's why pregnant women pee in a cup and submit to the blood pressure cuff so many times during checkups.

According to the National Institutes of Health, preeclampsia is the leading cause of maternal and fetal death in America. You may have rightly surmised from the "pre" in the name that there's also a condition called "eclampsia." It's a more severe form that can cause seizures, coma, and death, and it strikes one in two hundred women with preeclampsia.

The only real cure for preeclampsia is to deliver the baby, but if it pops up early in the pregnancy that may not be a feasible option.

The cause of preeclampsia is unknown, but doctors do know about the physical processes behind the condition, some of which make aspirin seem like a reasonable drug to use in preventing it.

For starters, the placenta—the structure connected to the wall of the woman's uterus that nourishes the fetus and removes its wastes—doesn't receive as much oxygen-rich blood as it should.

The mother's other organs begin receiving an inadequate amount of blood flow, her kidneys sustain damage, she gets inflammatory chemicals in her blood and in the placenta, and prostaglandins involved in her blood clotting get out of whack. Specifically, she creates too much thromboxane, which is a prostaglandin that causes increased clotting and blood-vessel tightness, and she runs comparatively low on prostacyclin, a counterbalancing prostaglandin that promotes dilation of blood vessels and less clotting.

Aspirin could conceivably be useful in preeclampsia by restoring a healthy balance between thromboxane and prostacyclin. As you've learned numerous times in this book, aspirin prevents the production of prostaglandins by inhibiting an enzyme—the COX enzyme—needed to make them.

Thromboxane is made by platelets in the bloodstream; once aspirin takes away their ability to make thromboxane, it doesn't return for the rest of the platelets' ten-day life. Only the new platelets that your body turns out afterward can clot. However, prostacyclin is mostly made by cells in the lining of your blood vessels, and they seem to be able to constantly make the COX enzyme, since they can begin making prostacyclin again after a dose of aspirin. Thus, taking aspirin daily seems to lower the amount of thromboxane more compared to the prostacyclin.

However, some major studies examining the use of aspirin to prevent preeclampsia have failed to lend support for widespread use of the drug.

In 1994, a randomized trial reported in the journal *Lancet* gave more than 9,000 pregnant women either low-dose aspirin or a placebo. The use of aspirin was associated with a small decrease in the number of women with preeclampsia marked by protein in their urine, but it wasn't statistically significant. However, they found that the low-dose aspirin was "generally safe" for the fetus and newborn baby. The authors surmised that the study didn't support the use of aspirin in *all* women at higher risk of preeclampsia, but it may be justified in women whose early preeclampsia would put them at a high risk of needing an early delivery.

In another study, reported in a 1998 *New England Journal of Medicine,* researchers gave low-dose aspirin or a placebo to more than

2,500 women who, for various reasons, faced a high chance of developing preeclampsia. The aspirin turned out to not significantly reduce the risk of preeclampsia.

However, some experts still find reason to believe that aspirin has benefits for women at high risk of developing the condition. In 2004, the Cochrane Collaboration—a well-known international organization that reviews medical literature to promote medical treatments that are supported by the best evidence—took a look at aspirin in preeclampsia.

After processing fifty-one trials involving more than 36,000 women, the reviewers found that anti-platelet drugs were associated with a 19 percent smaller risk of preeclampsia. They surmised that "antiplatelet agents (which were generally low-dose aspirin) have small to moderate benefits when used for the prevention of preeclampsia," but more information needs to be found out regarding which women will get the most benefit from it.

A similar meta-analysis, published in *Obstetrics & Gynecology* in 2003, combined the results of fourteen trials involving more than 12,000 women. It found that aspirin was associated with a 14 percent lower risk of preeclampsia. The authors concluded that "it seems reasonable to recommend aspirin therapy to women who are historically at high risk for preeclampsia, particularly those with multiple risk factors." These women at higher risk include those who had severe or early-onset preeclampsia in previous pregnancies, women with chronic high blood pressure, severe diabetes, or moderate to severe kidney disease.

Also, aspirin is a common treatment for women with a condition called antiphospholipid syndrome (APS), which can lead to preeclampsia. It's frequently combined with heparin, another anticlotting drug, to treat the condition, which can cause pregnancy loss due to improper blood flow to the placenta.

Neither of the two previous studies found harmful effects to the fetus from aspirin. The authors of the latter paper also reviewed the medical literature for large studies on the safety of aspirin in pregnancy. They found no evidence of birth defects or long-term harm to the baby from using aspirin while pregnant, though one study suggested a higher risk of miscarriage from NSAIDs used in the first twelve weeks of pregnancy.

However, you still *must* talk to your doctor before using aspirin if you're pregnant. The Food and Drug Administration suggests that women avoid the drug during the last three months of pregnancy unless under a doctor's advisement; high-dose aspirin in the last trimester may lead to a prolonged pregnancy and its accompanied risk of problems from the placenta no longer working properly.

In the Meantime, to Prevent Preeclampsia . . .

Making some lifestyle changes before you get pregnant may be more effective in preventing high blood pressure during pregnancy than aspirin, says Ronald F. Feinberg, M.D., Ph.D., the IVF medical director at Reproductive Associates of Delaware and author of *Healing Syndrome O: A Strategic Guide to Fertility, Polycystic Ovaries, and Insulin Imbalance* (Avery, 2004). Here are his recommendations:

- *Try to get yourself to a healthy weight before you become pregnant through a healthy diet and exercise routine.* Being obese going into a pregnancy may make you ten times more likely to have high blood pressure while you're pregnant
- *Give your body the best chance to use its insulin properly before you get pregnant.* Insulin resistance—a growing problem in America in which your body doesn't respond to a hormone used to usher blood sugar into cells after you eat—has been linked to high blood pressure in pregnancy in many studies. Regular exercise and a diet high in fiber and low in processed starches and sugars can help make you less likely to have insulin resistance.

MAKING A BETTER FERTILIZATION CONNECTION WITH ASPIRIN

In vitro fertilization, or IVF, is a form of assisted reproduction in which science takes over when the natural process isn't working. Couples may choose IVF when they can't conceive normally because the woman's fallopian tubes are blocked or she has endometriosis, or the man has difficulty contributing enough sperm.

In IVF, specialists remove eggs from the woman's ovary with a needle, fertilize them with the man's sperm in the laboratory, and implant the resulting embryos back in the woman's uterus a few days later. Successfully bringing a baby into the world this way can cost tens of thousands of dollars, as well as significant emotional upheaval.

In a Swedish study from a 2004 issue of the journal *Fertility and Sterility,* researchers gave aspirin to some women at an IVF clinic and not others, compiling data on 1,380 cycles of IVF. They gave low-dose aspirin daily from the point that the embryo was transferred into the woman until she took a pregnancy test. They found that the odds of a woman in the aspirin group giving birth were 20 percent higher (though due to the results it was also statistically possible that the aspirin had a smaller or no effect).

Since the process is so expensive and time-consuming, the authors state that "Given the importance of every birth in IVF, especially when taking into account the limited number of IVF cycles that are normally performed in an individual woman, any treatment to improve birth rate is important."

Also, aspirin might be useful for women whose endometrial lining in the uterus is too thin when doctors give them medicine to trigger ovulation or prepare for an IVF treatment, says Ronald F. Feinberg, M.D., Ph.D., medical director of the IVF program at Reproductive Associates of Delaware. He and colleagues typically recommend aspirin to these patients. "There is some evidence that aspirin might improve blood flow and possibly chances of implantation in such women. Most fertility specialists are frustrated with this problem and generally haven't had a lot of success overcoming it," he says.

It should go without saying that if you're going to embark on IVF, you should carefully follow your doctor's instructions and discuss the possible role of aspirin in your individual case with the physician before taking it.

In the Meantime, for IVF Success . . .

Plenty of steps other than aspirin will help improve your chances of a successful in vitro fertilization:

- *Don't smoke.* That goes for both of you—smoking makes men less fertile and decreases a woman's chance of getting pregnant, and also increases her risk of miscarriage. Steer clear of illegal drugs before and during the IVF treatment, too (and during pregnancy).
- *Curtail your drinking.* Women should abstain from alcohol before and during her IVF treatment, and avoid drinking while she's pregnant. Men trying to impregnate their partners should drink moderately at most, since excessive drinking reduces male fertility.
- *Chill out.* Staying de-stressed is important for the woman, and having good emotional support can improve her chances of getting pregnant. Be sure you have a friend, family member, or counselor who can help talk you through this trying time.

OTHER POSSIBLE BENEFITS

Aspirin use during pregnancy has also been associated with some other delivery-day bonuses, such as decreased risk of early delivery and increased birth weight.

In a 2003 meta-analysis, Canadian researchers evaluated thirty-eight studies while looking into the effects of aspirin on the outcome of the newborn baby. Women who took aspirin had an 8 percent lower risk of having a pre-term delivery. The babies born to women treated with aspirin were also, on average, a tiny bit heavier. That's not to say that aspirin is helpful for every woman, but you may find it worth discussing with your doctor.

In addition, Dr. Feinberg also feels that women with a history of excessive blood clotting probably need to take aspirin and low molecular weight heparin—another anticlotting drug—during pregnancy.

Section VI

Additional
Interesting Uses

You've now learned how aspirin can help prevent the "big" diseases, like heart attack, stroke, and cancer. In the following section, you'll see that it has lots of other uses and potential uses, too, ranging from conditions that you may have never heard about to common, everyday maladies like headaches.

11

Other Conditions

So far in this book you've learned about how aspirin can help keep you safe from big diseases, like cancer, heart attack, and stroke, or how it might make a little bit of a difference in situations where you can use all the help you can get, like in getting pregnant with an in vitro fertilization procedure.

This chapter is a little different. The following pages will discuss the use of aspirin in conditions for which the research is very preliminary; in conditions in which its use seems small but interesting; and in conditions you've probably never heard of in which it plays an important role.

OSTEOPOROSIS

Your bones may seem hard and unchanging, the same from day to day as the legs on your kitchen table. But actually, special cells in your bones are constantly breaking down and building back the structures; the cells taking out old bone are called osteo*clasts,* and the cells laying down new bone are called osteo*blasts.*

About two million "bone remodeling units" are turning over about 5 percent of your skeleton at any given time. Funny what you learn while reading about aspirin, huh?

According to laboratory research, prostaglandins may stimulate bone formation—but they may also increase the efforts of the osteoclasts, promoting bone loss. So inhibiting prostaglandins—which is what aspirin does— might theoretically increase or decrease bone mineral density.

Making bones denser is of utmost importance during osteoporosis, a condition that largely affects postmenopausal women by causing their bones to become more fragile and likely to break. Studies investigating a link between aspirin and other NSAIDs and fractures and bone-mineral density in white menopausal women in the late 1990s found conflicting results.

A 2003 study led by researchers at the University of Tennessee looked into the issue by examining data on bone-mineral density and NSAID use in 2,853 older adults, divided in half between men and women, and blacks and whites.

They found that people who were currently using a combination of aspirin (which affects both the COX-1 and COX-2 enzymes involved in producing prostaglandins) along with NSAIDs with more of an effect on the COX-2 enzyme had 4.2 percent higher bone-mineral density at the whole-body level and 4.6 percent higher density in their hips.

The effect of aspirin on bone is "small but positive," says Laura Carbone, M.D., an associate professor of rheumatology at the University of Tennessee, who has an interest in metabolic bone disorders. She has investigated the relationship between aspirin, the COX enzyme, and bone-mineral density.

The aspirin could tilt the bone-remodeling cycle slightly toward keeping the bone from being broken down as much, she says. She doesn't recommend anyone start taking aspirin just to prevent or treat osteoporosis, but if you're already taking it for other purposes, you can take some comfort knowing that it might also be helping your bones.

CYTOMEGALOVIRUS

"Cytomegalovirus" has a nasty sound to it. Actually, it sounds like a creature that would attack Tokyo in an old monster movie. At any rate, it has the ring of a dreadful invader that you don't want to have in your body.

If you're forty or over, though, you probably already do. According to the Centers for Disease Control and Prevention, this virus infects between 50 and 85 percent of adults by this age. For most people, becoming infected doesn't pose an immediate threat. If it causes symptoms, they're usually like those that occur from mononucleosis, such as fever and sore throat. The virus then takes up residence for the rest of the person's life, but lies dormant.

But the virus, which is related to the herpes viruses, the chicken pox virus, and the Epstein-Barr virus, *can* cause severe trouble. If women become infected during pregnancy, it can cause birth defects and mental retardation in the child (or death). In people with improperly working immune systems, like those with AIDS, it can cause pneumonia, eye infections, and gastrointestinal disease.

It also, as scientists are learning, just might play a role in atherosclerosis, the buildup of fat, cholesterol, and other debris in the walls of arteries that sets the stage for heart disease. The idea of a virus or bacteria contributing to atherosclerosis is nothing new—it was tossed around more than one hundred years ago—but it's been gaining more attention in recent years.

Cytomegalovirus (CMV) is among the small number of microbes that scientists are investigating in this process. The virus could begin the steps leading to atherosclerosis by causing injury to the lining of the artery. The body's inflammatory response causes immune cells to migrate to the area, leading to a chain of events culminating in a plaque that juts out from the vessel wall, narrowing the vessel.

Studies published in 2000 found that 76 percent of patients with ischemic heart disease had detectible amounts of DNA from the virus in their arterial wall, and up to 53 percent of spots of atherosclerosis in people's carotid arteries also had DNA from the virus.

How can aspirin potentially help? According to a study published in 1998 in the journal *Circulation Research,* when CMV infects cells in the smooth muscle in arteries, it quickly generates free radicals, or altered oxygen molecules. These, in turn, turn on a protein that causes cells to produce inflammatory chemicals. The familiar enzyme COX-2, which aspirin disables, may play a role in the generation of free radicals.

So, in addition to its ability to make blood less likely to form clots in narrowed arteries, aspirin might also play a role in preventing heart disease by inhibiting atherosclerosis resulting from infection by this virus, the scientists reason.

KAWASAKI DISEASE

The most common cause of acquired heart disease in children is a condition you might not have even heard of before.

Kawasaki disease primarily affects children under the age of five. It's more likely to strike children of Asian—particularly Japanese—descent, and it's named after a Japanese physician.

Exactly what causes it is unknown, though it could be some sort of infectious organism, such as a virus or bacteria. The condition often starts with a high fever that may last five days or even a few weeks. Affected children's eyes and mouths may grow red, they may have swollen lymph nodes, and their skin may peel away, particularly on the palms of the hands and soles of the feet.

Even more worrisome, the condition can cause inflammation in the child's coronary arteries. This inflammation can cause weak, bulging spots in the arteries, where blood clots may form. Around 20 percent of children with Kawasaki disease have artery inflammation. The resulting clots may cause heart attacks, though this is rare.

One of the standard treatments for the disease is gamma globulin, which reduces inflammation and is given through a vein. The other is high doses of aspirin. The aspirin reduces the risk of blood clots. The child may need to continue on lower doses of aspirin for several weeks or months.

POLYCYTHEMIA VERA

Once or twice in his or her career, the average family doctor will diagnose a rare and serious blood disorder that often has an odd but specific symptom: The patient will feel itchy after a warm bath or shower.

This disorder, polycythemia vera, occurs when a person's bone marrow starts producing too many blood cells—particularly red blood cells, but also white blood cells and platelets. The name is a mini-lesson in ancient languages: Poly-cyt-hemia is Greek for "many, cells, and blood," while vera is Latin for "true," which distinguishes this disease from others with similar features whose causes are known. What causes polycythemia vera is unknown.

The condition makes a person's blood become thicker and sludgy, and often causes headache, dizziness, nosebleeds, and facial flushing. It most often occurs in people around the age of sixty.

Aside from these symptoms, the condition also causes life-threatening problems. People with the disease have a higher chance of complications from clotting, such as heart attacks and strokes. It may also progress to leukemia.

If untreated, people can expect to live only six to eighteen months after diagnosis. With treatment, patients may survive more than ten years.

The backbone of treatment for this disease is phlebotomy—in other words, regularly draining off blood. Also, a variety of medications are sometimes used to reduce bone-marrow activity. Another treatment—which has been controversial—is aspirin.

In the 1980s, high-dose aspirin was used with another drug that keeps platelets from sticking together—dipyridamole—but it caused too much bleeding in the gastrointestinal tract. Thus, it largely fell from favor for fifteen years or so, says Steven Fruchtman, M.D., a clinical associate professor at the Mount Sinai School of Medicine in New York and an expert on blood disorders.

However, more recent research from Europe looked at more than 1,600 people with the disease to get more details on how it progresses. Part of this research was a study that gave 518 of the subjects either low-dose aspirin or a placebo. The aspirin was associated with a 59 percent reduction in cardiovascular-related deaths. There was a slight increase in major bleeding, but it wasn't statistically significant.

Thus, a 2003 publication from the American Society of Hematology recommended the use of low-dose aspirin for the long-term management of the condition, except in people who clearly should avoid the drug.

Many physicians are now recommending a daily dose of "baby aspirin," or 81 milligrams, in addition to regular blood-drawing and, in many patients, drugs to reduce bone-marrow activity, Dr. Fruchtman says.

12

Everyday Uses

For much of the past one hundred years, before people ever knew that aspirin could protect them from fatal diseases, they took billions upon billions of aspirin for more mundane yet aggravating problems. Their heads throbbed, their fever raged, their joints screamed . . . and they reached for the trusty bottle of aspirin.

So even though you won't see many headlines in the news about these uses of aspirin, take a look at the following benefits of the drug to make sure you're using it to its maximum effectiveness.

HEADACHE

Here's some surprising news: According to the American Council on Headache Education, almost 90 percent of men and 95 percent of women had a headache during the past year. The surprising part of that fact is that some people didn't get a headache last year!

Until the rest of us learn the secret to a headache-free life, we can rely on aspirin to shoo the pain away. Aspirin is effective in treating two of the most common types of headaches, including the dreaded, disabling migraine. However, it's important to know how to use the drug to avoid bringing on even more headaches.

Tension Headache

The most common form of headache, according to the National Headache Foundation, are tension headaches, which seem to be linked to muscle tightness in the neck and scalp. They cause pain on both sides of the head, which in some sufferers feels like a band of pressure clamping down on the skull.

Tension headaches are divided into three categories, based on how often they occur. Episodic headaches strike less than once per month and may be brought on by stress or tiredness. Frequent tension headaches strike up to fifteen days per month. A chronic tension headache tends to linger constantly.

People generally treat tension headaches on their own with over-the-counter painkillers—and lots of them. Americans spend roughly $1 billion each year on these drugs for headache relief. Aspirin's effectiveness in treating tension headaches has been well-established by scientific studies. It's more effective for headaches than acetaminophen, according to *Management of Headache and Headache Medications* by Lawrence D. Robbins, M.D.

Aspirin helps relieve tension headaches by reducing prostaglandins, which make your nerve endings more sensitive to pain.

Doses between 500 and 1,000 milligrams have been shown to relieve tension-headache pain within sixty minutes. The usual dose for headaches is 325 to 650 milligrams every four hours as needed in adults, and 325 milligrams every four to six hours as needed in children (but don't give it to them if they may have the flu or chicken pox).

Caffeine adds to aspirin's effectiveness, aiding in its pain-relieving power, which is why several over-the-counter headache remedies include caffeine. If you don't have one of these brands handy and would like the caffeine boost, have a cup of coffee or several cups of tea with your aspirin. However, be sure to read the section on "rebound headaches" later in the chapter, as aspirin and caffeine overuse can lead to these.

Migraine

If you're feeling a migraine coming on, your best bet may be to head to the nearest bottle of aspirin. The U.S. Headache Consortium, a group of seven health organizations that deal with migraine treatment, recommends aspirin and other over-the-counter NSAIDs as a good first-line treatment for mild to moderate migraines, or even severe migraines if the drugs have eased them before.

This includes the combination of aspirin with caffeine and acetaminophen, which is found in Excedrin. In 1998, the Food and Drug Administration approved changing the label on Excedrin to make it the first over-the-counter product specifically for treating migraines.

Migraines affect more than twenty-five million Americans; they're three times more common in women than in men. They may be triggered by bright or flickering lights, certain foods, altered sleep or eating patterns, and stress.

The pain from migraine is usually a moderate to severe throbbing sensation focused on one side of the head. People with migraines may also be nauseous and sensitive to light. Many people with migraines first see an "aura," or a sparkly or fuzzy area in their field of vision, several minutes before the migraine starts.

Aspirin may help relieve migraine pain by reducing production of prostaglan-

What exactly is going on in your head during a migraine is still something of a mystery. Experts think the complicated process involves the trigeminal nerve in the head becoming overstimulated, which causes blood vessels around the brain to become dilated, inflamed, and painful. The overstimulation of the trigeminal nerve may be caused by a brain chemical called serotonin, released when platelets in the blood clump together.

dins, as well as keeping platelets from clumping and reducing serotonin release.

According to an overview of over-the-counter drugs for migraine published in the journal *Pharmacotherapy* in 2003, up to three-fourths of people can "return to normal functioning" within two hours of taking aspirin; people with less-severe attacks have the best chance of quick relief. Some people can even be pain-free within two hours.

In his book, Dr. Robbins recommends Extra Strength Excedrin, also known as Excedrin Migraine, as a first-line medication to treat a migraine in adults, at a dosage of one or two tablets every three hours as needed.

For children, he recommends aspirin as a second-tier choice due to concerns about Reye's syndrome (see page 168 for more on this issue). For ages six to eight, give a dose of 325 milligrams every four hours as needed, and at age nine and ten, give 400 milligrams every four hours. To make the medication more effective with caffeine, give Anacin, which contains caffeine, or let the child wash down the aspirin with a soda.

Rebound Headache

Be careful not to use aspirin too frequently to deal with headache pain (either tension or migraines); ironically, overuse of over-the-counter pain relievers can actually *cause* chronic headaches. This is a particular risk from brands containing caffeine, which several aspirin-based pain relievers contain.

According to the National Headache Foundation, people may unwittingly get into a routine in which they use their headache medicine more than the label recommends, which leads to even more headaches. This, in turn, causes the person to take even more medication more frequently.

These rebound headaches are often associated with waking up early with a headache, nausea, restlessness, depression, poor appetite and difficulty concentrating. The NHF suggests that if you're using headache medications more than two days a week, you may be overusing them. Consider visiting your doctor to look into other medications or non-drug steps such as smoking cessation, if you smoke, and relaxation techniques.

ARTHRITIS

NSAIDs, including aspirin, have long played an important role in reducing pain and inflammation in arthritis. The drugs work by reducing prostaglandins in the body that promote inflammation and pain.

The two most common forms of arthritis are osteoarthritis, in which cartilage in the joints dwindles, allowing the ends of bones to rub together; and rheumatoid arthritis, marked by damaging inflammation in the joints.

Osteoarthritis is most common in older people and typically strikes weight-bearing joints like the hips and knees, as well as the hands. Obesity and certain physical professions and activities may increase the risk of the condition.

Rheumatoid arthritis, on the other hand, most commonly strikes between the ages of thirty and fifty, most often women. It brings inflammation, pain, and swelling in the joints.

Until recent times, doctors started patients with rheumatoid arthritis on NSAIDs and only moved on to other treatments once the disease had gotten worse, according to the Arthritis Foundation. However, doctors now start prescribing drugs called disease-modifying antirheumatic drugs (DMARDs) earlier in the disease to slow or prevent permanent joint damage and disability.

However, aspirin and other NSAIDs still offer important benefits in rheumatoid arthritis. No NSAID has been shown to work consistently better than others for rheumatoid arthritis; individuals may have to experiment to find the one that works best for them. However, aspirin has been shown to be on the low end of causing gastrointestinal damage, as far as NSAIDs are concerned. It's also inexpensive, which can be an important factor, considering the amount of aspirin needed to control symptoms.

If you use aspirin to control your arthritis, you're probably going to be taking significant doses of it. The Arthritis Foundation recommends 2,400 to 5,400 milligrams daily in divided doses to keep symptoms in check. Aspirin can cause side effects—which typically start with reversible deafness or ringing in the ears—at high doses, so be sure to work with your doctor to find the dose that works for you.

DENTAL PAIN

Forget about aspirin being a "mild analgesic" for dental pain, as medical experts sometimes call it. Doses of aspirin of more than 500 milligrams have been found to have at least as much pain-relieving power as the amount of the narcotic codeine found in two Tylenol with Codeine #3 or the amount of oxycodone found in one Percocet.

However, the drug is intended to go down your throat—not stay in your mouth. Never hold an aspirin against your tooth or gum. Contact with aspirin can burn your gums and damage the enamel that covers your teeth.

MENSTRUAL PAIN

If you're a woman whose cycle brings a monthly round of menstrual cramping, aspirin could be a powerful tool to put a crimp on the cramps. Prostaglandins seem to be a major cause of cramps, and aspirin blocks the production of these hormone-like chemicals.

A meta-analysis—or research project that compiles the results of multiple studies on a topic—looked into the effects of aspirin on menstrual pain and found that doses between 500 and 650 milligrams four times daily were significantly more effective than a placebo.

Section VII

Reducing Complications of Aspirin Use

Nothing in life is completely safe, and aspirin is no exception. While we'd like such a useful medication to only give us benefits without causing any side effects, that's just not possible.

However, it *is* possible to protect yourself from aspirin's potential side effects. By working with your doctor, you may still be able to take aspirin while preventing damage to your stomach and intestine. You may even be able to take aspirin if it's previously caused your asthma to flare up. You'll learn how in the following pages.

You'll also learn in this section more about how to take aspirin safely and avoid side effects caused by taking it with the wrong medications or herbs.

13

Reducing the Risk
of Complications

 A doctor who's trained to peer inside a person's belly with an endoscope can see how aspirin quickly starts causing effects . . . but not in a good way.

After someone has taken aspirin for a few days—even in low doses—the doctor will likely see "a constellation" of minor injuries while peering through the endoscope into his or her stomach, says Byron Cryer, M.D., a gastroenterologist and associate professor of internal medicine at the University of Texas Southwestern Medical School, who studies the effects of NSAIDs on the stomach.

About 90 percent of people taking aspirin will have erosions, or areas of superficial etching into the lining of the stomach, and *petechial hemorrhages,* or pinpoint-sized bleeding spots, after a few days of regular use, Dr. Cryer says.

"That's the bad news," he says. However, these little injuries generally don't cause any symptoms, nor do they predict who will go on to have more serious problems from aspirin, he says. In other words, the erosions and pinprick bleeding spots aren't a big concern. That's good news.

Plus, "The upside of the discussion is with continued exposure to aspirin, the stomach becomes somewhat resilient to the development of these minor degrees of injury," he says. If the doctor were to inspect the lining of your stomach three months after you've been taking aspirin regularly, your stomach would likely have adapted to the drug, and you'd show far fewer signs of damage in the lining.

However, a small percentage of people who use aspirin and other NSAIDs will have serious gastrointestinal side effects of the medications, including peptic ulcers. These are spots in the stomach and duodenum—the first part of the small intestine—where acid has caused damage in the organs' lining. These ulcers can go all the way through the wall of the organ.

Prostaglandins help protect the mucous lining of the stomach and duodenum from their harsh environment, possibly by stimulating secretion of protective bicarbonate and mucus, increasing blood flow, and increasing the proliferation of cells in the lining. However, aspirin decreases the production of these protective prostaglandins, leaving the gastrointestinal tract less defended.

Signs of bleeding related to ulcers include vomiting blood, a black, tarry stool—which indicates digested blood—or red blood in the stool, says Jay Goldstein, M.D., a professor of medicine at the University of Illinois at Chicago, whose research interests include the role of NSAIDs in stomach and small-intestine ulcers.

A Spanish study, reported in 2001, compared 2,105 cases of upper gastrointestinal bleeding or perforation to 11,500 healthy people without these problems, and compared the people's exposure to aspirin. It found that people exposed to aspirin had twice the risk of these problems as people who hadn't taken the drug.

Although enteric-coated aspirin, which is sheathed in ingredients that allow the drug to get past the stomach before dissolving, is intended to reduce stomach discomfort from the drug, the study didn't see a difference between plain and enteric-coated aspirin in regards to these complications.

However, if you find yourself with dyspepsia, or stomach discomfort, after you've begun an aspirin regimen, coated aspirin should reduce your discomfort, Dr. Cryer says.

Although doubling your risk of something unpleasant is always a scary thought, keep in mind that the majority of people who take aspirin won't have one of these events. A 2000 meta-analysis from the *British Medical Journal* pooled the results of twenty-four other studies that compared the number of gastrointestinal hemorrhages in people taking aspirin for more than a year versus the number in those who took a placebo or no treatment.

It found that about 1 percent of people taking aspirin over a 28-month period will have gastrointestinal bleeding (it didn't specify the severity of the event). The risk of complications is highest during the first few months of taking the drug.

Factors that increase the chance of having bleeding include advanced age—the older you are, the more likely you'll have a problem—and having a history of previous peptic ulcers.

However, by working with your doctor you can reduce your risk of gastrointestinal bleeding. You can also reduce your chances of having bleeding in your brain, which is another complication associated with taking aspirin. And if you have asthma and other allergic symptoms after taking aspirin, a simple procedure can allow you to take the drug without harm.

PROTECTING YOUR BELLY FROM HARM

One of the leading causes of peptic ulcers is NSAID use, which includes aspirin. But the most common cause is infection from the *Helicobacter pylori* germ. Making sure you don't have it in your belly before you start taking long-term aspirin can decrease your chances of gastrointestinal complications.

Most people who harbor the germ in their stomachs don't develop peptic ulcers—which is good, since so many of us have it. According to the National Institutes of Health, about 20 percent of people under forty years old are carrying around *H. pylori,* a figure that rises to half of people over the age of sixty. It may spread through food and water, and kissing.

The germ is able to live in the acidic environment of the stomach, and it can burrow into the mucous lining that protects the organ from acid. The acid and the bacteria damage the lining, causing an ulcer.

During the 1990s, some studies showed increased damage from NSAIDs in people with *H. pylori* infection, but others showed opposite results, or no relationship. However, more recent studies have shown that *H. pylori* aids in the development of injury to the mucous lining from low-dose aspirin.

In a 2002 study from Spain, 98 people with upper gastrointestinal bleeding who had taken low-dose aspirin were compared to 147 people without bleeding who had taken low-dose aspirin. Being infected with *H. pylori* was determined to make people taking low-dose aspirin almost five times more likely to bleed.

As a result, some doctors recommend that patients who are at high risk of digestive bleeding from aspirin be tested for the germ before beginning aspirin therapy, Dr. Cryer says. He makes this recommendation himself.

People at high risk include those who have had a previous ulcer or gastrointestinal bleeding, he says. Other factors that some experts point out will put you at higher risk include old age, use of high-dose or multiple NSAIDs, and using aspirin along with other antiplatelet drugs or warfarin (Coumadin).

However, some experts recommend that *anyone* who's about to start a regimen of low-dose aspirin for their cardiovascular health first be tested for *H. pylori* and get treated if necessary. So should anyone who's currently taking long-term aspirin therapy and has a history of indigestion or peptic ulcer.

Doctors can diagnose *H. pylori* infection through simple means such as testing your blood from a pinprick to check for antibodies you may be producing against the bacteria; checking your breath after you swallow a special solution to look for signs of *H. pylori* activity; and examining a sample of your stool for signs of the bacteria.

For most people, getting rid of the bug is a simple process that takes only two weeks, Dr. Cryer says. Eradication requires a combination of antibiotics along with an acid-reducing medication called a proton-pump inhibitor (PPI). These are effective in clearing away *H. pylori* in about 80 percent of people, he says.

A PPI also can play a longer-running role in protecting your stomach while you're taking aspirin, particularly if you're at high risk due to your age, a history of ulcers, or if you take multiple NSAIDs, or aspirin in conjunction with other anti-clotting drugs or steroids.

These medications have been found to reduce the risk of ulcers, and a number of experts on gastrointestinal damage from NSAIDs have recommended them for higher-risk patients as part of an ulcer-prevention strategy.

PPIs—a well-known one of which is esoneprazole (Nexium)—prevent cells in the stomach from secreting hydrochloric acid. These drugs have been shown to be more effective in preventing ulcers related to NSAIDs than the drugs known as H_2 blockers, such as Pepcid, Tagamet, and Zantac, which also work to reduce acid in the stomach.

Another drug that's been shown to reduce the chances of ulcer problems while you're taking NSAIDs is misoprostol (Cytotec). In fact, research has shown it to be even more effective in protecting patients from ulcers than a PPI while they're taking NSAIDs. The drug is a synthetic version of a prostaglandin, and it can help protect the stomach in a variety of ways, such as by increasing the production of protective mucus and bicarbonate in the stomach and reducing acid secretion.

However, people often walk away from the drug's benefits because of the side effects it causes—namely, diarrhea.

If you're regularly taking aspirin for a problem with no symptoms (such as preventing heart attack or stroke), you're unlikely to want to take a medicine that carries unpleasant side effects, Dr. Cryer says. Thus, chances are you'll find misoprostol unappealing. However, it's worth talking to your doctor about it when you discuss ways to prevent gastrointestinal complications of aspirin, since it doesn't give everyone diarrhea. Note: Women who are pregnant should avoid the drug.

Protect Yourself from Brain Bleeding While on Aspirin

As you learned earlier in the book, taking regular aspirin can make you slightly more likely to have a hemorrhagic stroke. This causes bleeding in the brain, and the consequences can be deadly.

The increased risk of this complication is a major reason why doctors aren't enthusiastic to put more people on aspirin for protection against heart attacks and another type of stroke.

However, if you're going to take long-term aspirin, you can take steps to reduce your risk of hemorrhagic stroke. The most important steps are making sure your blood pressure is under good control and avoiding smoking.

According to the National Heart, Lung, and Blood Institute, your blood pressure is considered high—a condition called hypertension—once it reaches 140/90 mmHg. Anything between 120/80 and 139/89 mmHg is considered *pre*hypertension.

Getting your blood pressure to a healthy level involves working with your doctor, who will want to check your pressure regularly. The following approaches will help lower your blood pressure:

- Losing weight if you're overweight.
- Getting thirty minutes of physical activity most days of the week.
- Eating a diet that's high in fruits, vegetables, whole grains, and low-fat dairy. Most Americans consume too much sodium, and you need to be sure you keep sodium limited in your diet.
- Taking one or more blood pressure–lowering medications.
- Drinking alcohol in moderation, at most.

Also, if you smoke, talk to your doctor about ways to stop. Nicotine raises your blood pressure, and smoking increases your risk of ischemic stroke, which is much more common than hemorrhagic stroke.

REDUCING BREATHING
COMPLICATIONS FROM ASTHMA

In some people, aspirin's most noticeable effect isn't relief from pain and inflammation. Instead, within a few minutes or hours after popping an aspirin, some people develop a stuffy nose, wheezing, and difficulty breathing. These symptoms can be merely annoying, but can also be dangerous.

Aspirin-induced breathing problems may be a serious problem for many people with asthma. A 2004 study in the *British Medical Journal,* which reviewed a number of other papers that measured the prevalence of aspirin-induced asthma, found that 21 percent of adults with asthma and 5 percent of children with the condition have worsened symptoms when they take aspirin. Some other studies, however, have put the number lower.

People with asthma-induced allergy also often have nasal polyps, which are noncancerous growths in the nose that are removed surgically.

According to a 2004 issue of the *Harvard Heart Letter,* the problem stems from aspirin's ability to block the activity of the COX enzyme. This enzyme is used in the body to convert a substance called arachidonic acid into hormonelike chemicals called prostaglandins. Aspirin disables the COX-1 enzyme, thereby leaving more arachidonic acid unconverted. According to the publication, people who are allergic to aspirin then turn the unused arachidonic acid into compounds called leukotrienes. These promote inflammation in the airways, constrict air-carrying tubes in the lungs, promote mucus secretion in the airways, and cause tissues in the nose to swell.

Aspirin isn't the only medication that triggers these problems. People with the condition also have symptoms after taking other NSAIDs, such as ibuprofen (Advil), ketoprofen (Orudis), and naproxen (Aleve). Acetaminophen, which is found in Tylenol, relieves pain but doesn't trigger these problems at normal dosages, since it only weakly acts on COX-1. COX-2 inhibitors, such as Celebrex, aren't thought to cause these problems, either.

However, even if you have asthma symptoms triggered by aspirin, you can undergo a simple procedure to desensitize yourself to the drug if you want to take it for its health-promoting benefits.

In one well-known method, the "Scripps Clinic Protocol," you take three doses of placebo spaced three hours apart on the first day. The second day, you take 30 milligrams of aspirin, then three hours later take 45 to 60, then three hours later take 60 to 100. On the third day, you take 100 to 150, 150 to 325, and 325 to 650 milligrams spaced three hours apart.

This is all done in an allergist's office where the staff can monitor you and quickly treat you in case an emergency arises. If you reach a dose that causes symptoms, you repeat it until it doesn't cause problems.

After you reach the highest amount, you're set. After that, you must take some aspirin every day, even if just a low dose of 81 milligrams. If you miss several days, your symptoms will return again when you take an aspirin.

14

Warnings

Despite the ease with which most of us toss it back without much thought, aspirin is indeed a drug. Like other drugs, it's possible to overdose on it, and it can interact harmfully with other drugs and herbs. In some instances, you should talk to your doctor before taking it or giving it to a family member, and in some instances aspirin should be avoided.

Here's a rundown of some particulars you need to know to make sure aspirin does you and your family the most good.

OVERDOSING

It's possible to overdose on aspirin if you take a huge dose at one time (called *acute* salicylate intoxication), or regularly exceed a wise dosage (called *chronic* salicylate intoxication).

People have died from taking 10 to 30 grams—that's 10,000 to 30,000 milligrams—in one fell swoop. That's at least thirty regular-strength aspirin, which you're unlikely to take by accident.

It may also be possible for, say, a 150-pound person to have chronic salicylate intoxication, also called *salicylism,* from taking 6,800 milligrams a day for two days or more. That greatly exceeds the recommended adult dosage for preventing heart disease, and even exceeds the recommended dosage for arthritis. However, a smaller person wouldn't need to take as much to have side effects.

In adults, the most common symptoms of chronic salicylate intoxication is ringing of the ears and hearing loss. Other symptoms include drowsiness, confusion, dizziness, lethargy, vomiting, thirst, and hyperventilation. In children the most frequent symptoms are hyperventilation, giddiness, drowsiness, and behavioral changes.

If you think you or someone else might have overdosed on aspirin, contact emergency medical help. Depending on the severity, doctors may need to induce vomiting, pump your stomach, and treat you with fluids and dialysis.

HERB/DRUG INTERACTIONS

Some things are meant to go together, like peanut butter and jelly. Aspirin, however, often likes to travel alone. In the following cases, taking these drugs or other substances along with aspirin could reduce their effectiveness or cause harm. Be sure to talk to your doctor before taking aspirin, particularly in high doses or for extended periods, if you're taking the following:

- *Alcohol.* Alcohol increases the likelihood and severity of GI bleeding caused by aspirin, so you should avoid consuming alcohol close to when you take aspirin. If you generally consume three or more alcoholic drinks daily, talk to your doctor about whether you should take aspirin.
- *Antacids.* Chronic use of antacids, such as citrates, sodium bicarbonate, and antacids with calcium or magnesium, can cause you to excrete more of the aspirin you take in your urine, mak-

ing it less effective. Similarly, stopping regular antacid use if you're taking regular aspirin may make your body's salicylate level rise too high.

- *Beta-blockers.* Aspirin may make these blood pressure–lowering drugs less effective.
- *Diabetes drugs.* Taking aspirin in high doses may increase the effectiveness of insulin and other diabetes drugs.
- *Drugs harmful to the ears.* High doses of aspirin can cause reversible hearing loss, and you should avoid aspirin when taking drugs that can cause hearing damage. The combination can cause *permanent* hearing loss. These drugs include—but aren't limited to—furosemide (Lasix), a diuretic; and vancomycin, an antibiotic.
- *Foods with salicylates.* While taking aspirin, limit your intake of prunes, raisins, tea, gherkins, Benedictine liqueur, curry powder, paprika, and licorice. All contain salicylates, and could lead to excessive salicylate accumulation in your body.
- *Gout medications.* Aspirin isn't recommended if you're taking probenecid (Benemid) or sulfinpyrazone (Anturan), which are used for treating gout. It may decrease their effectiveness.
- *Herbs and drugs with antiplatelet effect.* Aspirin prevents platelets in your blood from sticking together, thereby making your blood less likely to clot. Taking aspirin with other antiplatelet drugs such as clopidogrel (Plavix); or anticoagulants such as warfarin (Coumadin) and heparin may increase your bleeding time.

    Avoid taking herbs with antiplatelet effects while taking aspirin. These include garlic, ginkgo, ginger, ginseng, green tea, horse chestnut, feverfew, red clover, dong quai, and cat's claw.
- *Methotrexate.* Aspirin can cause toxic buildup of this drug used for treating cancer, psoriasis, and arthritis. If you're taking aspirin, your methotrexate dosage should be lowered, and you should discontinue aspirin at least a day before undergoing a large-dose infusion of methotrexate.
- *Other NSAIDs.* Taking aspirin along with other nonsteroidal anti-inflammatory drugs (NSAIDs), both over-the-counter and

prescription, may increase your risk of ulcers and bleeding in your gastrointestinal tract. It may also increase your risk of bleeding elsewhere in your body.

- *Tetracyclines.* Taking buffered aspirin may decrease your body's absorption of these drugs, which are used to treat acne and infections.
- *Valproic acid.* Taking aspirin with this anti-epilepsy drug, also known as Depakote, may increase your chance of bleeding.

OTHER CONTRAINDICATIONS

The following situations may also make aspirin an inappropriate choice:

- *Bleeding disorders.* People with conditions causing excessive bleeding should avoid aspirin. These include hemophilia, vitamin K deficiency, hypoprothrombinemia, and thrombocytopenia.
- *Impaired kidney function.* If your kidneys aren't working properly, approach aspirin with caution, since your kidneys are almost totally responsible for excreting the aspirin out of your body. You're also at increased risk of kidney damage from aspirin.
- *Pre-surgery.* Aspirin affects platelets and makes them less likely to form clots for more than a week. In general, you should stop taking aspirin for a week or so before surgery to decrease your risk of excessive bleeding. However, talk to your doctor before discontinuing aspirin.
- *Oral surgery.* Avoid chewing gum containing aspirin, or chewable aspirin, for at least a week after tonsillectomy or oral surgery. The aspirin may cause injury to sensitive tissues in the area or make blood vessels bleed.

REYE'S SYNDROME

Most of this book examines the use of aspirin to prevent diseases that are largely the burden of adults, like heart disease and stroke, so it's not really directed at the teen-and-under crowd. But aspirin *has* been used for reducing fevers in kids, which isn't a good idea, for the following reason:

Reye's syndrome is a condition with an unknown cause, but it's linked to taking aspirin at the wrong time. Though it can affect adults, it's largely a problem found in children and teens who take aspirin or other salicylates during a fever.

It typically occurs about a week after the patient has had an upper-respiratory infection, such as the flu, or chicken pox; cases have shown up in increased numbers during the winter months. The condition is marked by fatigue, vomiting, and lethargy, which can progress to coma and death. Organs that are particularly affected by Reye's are the liver, which develops fatty accumulation, and the brain, which swells.

Thankfully, reports of Reye's have fallen dramatically since 1980, when more than 550 cases were reported. By the late 1990s, annual reported cases had fallen into the single digits. This may be due to fewer children taking aspirin and similar products, as well as doctors properly diagnosing cases of metabolic diseases with similar symptoms that once would have been called Reye's.

To reduce the chances of Reye's affecting your household, avoid giving aspirin or related drugs to children or teens unless advised by a physician. Be particularly careful to avoid using these medications during a fever. These drugs include salicylates, too, so be sure to check the package carefully for more than just the word "aspirin." Pepto-Bismol, for example, contains bismuth subsalicylate and should be avoided in these cases.

Section VIII

The Future
of Aspirin

In coming years, aspirin may become even better than it already is. Researchers are seeking ways to make the drug safer for your stomach, as well as ways to make it into new shapes and textures so it can be painted onto surgical implants to help prevent complications they can cause.

15

New Forms of Aspirin

Aspirin is surprisingly lively and active, considering it's been around for more than a century. However, even something that remains relevant after one hundred years can benefit from a makeover. Researchers around the world are tinkering with aspirin in hopes of making it useful for more applications, with fewer harmful effects on the body.

Here are some aspirin-related developments you might see in the news in coming years:

WHEN NO IS A GOOD WORD

Bayer discovered it had a blockbuster drug on its hands after it chemically added acetic acid to a popular anti-inflammatory drug of the day, salicylic acid, to form aspirin. A French company is now looking into whether adding another chemical can make aspirin safer.

The company, NicOx, has been investigating a drug it calls NCX-4016 (hopefully they'll think of a catchier name if they bring it to the market). It's a form of aspirin that releases nitric oxide. According to the *Harvard Health Letter,* nitric oxide (abbreviated NO) in the body helps immune cells fight off infection, it helps blood vessels stay supple, and it may help protect the stomach by increasing blood flow to its walls.

In preclinical studies, researchers found that NCX-4016 had the helpful abilities of aspirin, such as its anti-inflammatory, pain-relieving, and anticlotting effects, but was "virtually devoid" of gastrointestinal toxicity. As you know, an unfortunate effect of aspirin is that it can cause gastrointestinal damage, which is a major reason it's not more widely used. Even the prescription anti-inflammatory drugs called COX-2 inhibitors, which in theory should avoid causing this damage since they work differently from aspirin, can still have this effect.

In a 2003 study from Italy, researchers divided forty healthy men and women into five groups. Twice a day for a week they either took a higher or lower dose of regular aspirin, a higher or lower dose of NCX-4016, or a placebo. Investigators inspected all the subjects' stomachs and first section of their small intestines before and after, and measured their blood's ability to clot.

They found that the new drug interfered with the clotting ability of the subjects' platelets equally as well as aspirin did, while causing hardly any gastrointestinal damage.

The drug has also been shown in research to offer protection to the stomach when taken along with aspirin. In a 2004 study, also from Italy, researchers split forty-eight adults into four groups. For twenty-one days they took either NCX-4016 twice a day; NCX-4016 plus aspirin twice a day; just aspirin; or just placebo.

Those who took the new drug plus the aspirin had less gastrointestinal injury than the people who took just the aspirin.

As of late 2004, the company had shown that the drug has a statistically significant effect in treating blood-vessel dysfunction in people with peripheral arterial disease and was engaged in another study investigating whether the drug would help people with this condition be able to walk farther. It expected to announce the results sometime in 2005.

Other nitric oxide–added versions of drugs the company is investigating include acetaminophen (the drug in Tylenol); hydrocortisone, a steroid cream for treating skin inflammation; an antihistamine for hay fever; flurbiprofen (a prescription NSAID); and budesonide, a corticosteroid allergy drug.

"Plastic" Aspirin

A chemical known as styrene is normally found in liquid form. But when you take several molecules of styrene and put them into a structure called a polymer, they form a solid material known as polystyrene. You may know this material as Styrofoam, which is used to make coffee cups.

Another well-known name for a polymer is plastic, points out Kathryn Uhrich, Ph.D., a chemist and associate professor at Rutgers University in New Jersey. Dr. Uhrich has been working in recent years to develop aspirin derivatives into a polymer form, a substance she calls PolyAspirin. It's made of molecules of salicylic acid, an ingredient of aspirin, combined with a fatty acid.

If you drop PolyAspirin into a glass of water, it won't rapidly dissolve like aspirin does. If a person were to take it, it wouldn't break down in the stomach, either, but would dissolve in the intestine, releasing its salicylic acid. However, Dr. Uhrich isn't investigating the drug's use for problems such as headaches.

Instead, she sees PolyAspirin as a useful coating for devices surgically implanted in the body. For example, stents are little metallic tubes that surgeons put into narrowed arteries to hold them open so blood can flow through them. A possible complication, though, is that blood clots can form on the stents. Aspirin and other anticlotting drugs are recommended for people after they get stents implanted to prevent clots.

A PolyAspirin coating on a stent could slowly dissolve, putting the drug only where it needs to be instead of distributing it through the body like a regular aspirin. This could conceivably prevent re-narrowing of the artery near the device, she says.

"We're also exploring using the plastic as a coating that you could paint onto orthopedic implants, such as hip implants," she says. "It'll only be there temporarily, but in that interim period, presumably it would help reduce inflammation and pain."

The material can be formed into a variety of different textures for different uses, and the speed at which it breaks down can also be controlled, she says.

"Do you want something like chewing gum or something more brittle like a CD disc? Do you want something transparent? Do you want something that can bend very easily or something stiff? We can manipulate it," she says.

She's formed a company, Polymerix, to develop the polymer aspirin, as well as a number of other NSAIDs and other drugs in polymer form. The company has already conducted preclinical testing on the substance and has sought the FDA's approval to begin testing the product in clinical trials, possibly in the spring of 2005.

Appendix: Types of Aspirin and Their Uses

Your doctor and pharmacist can provide you with several medications that combine aspirin with other drugs in prescription form to treat a number of ailments.

In one drug, aspirin is combined with a nervous-system relaxant to treat headaches. In another it's combined with a drug for relieving anxiety and tension. In yet another it's combined with a muscle relaxant for treating strains.

However, you'll find an even greater variety of types of aspirin out on the shelves that are available without a prescription. They come in many dosages and formulations, allowing you to chew the aspirin, drink it, or go a different route entirely and insert it as a suppository.

The following information will discuss the types of aspirin you may come across and the benefits and shortcomings each may have. This list is based on brands and dosages based in America, but it's not exhaustive.

Enteric-Coated

Aspirin Regimen Bayer—81 mg, 325 mg
Ecotrin—81 mg, 325 mg, 500 mg
St. Joseph—81 mg

You may also see these called "safety coated" on the package. "Enteric" refers to the small intestine, where these break down in the alkaline environment, rather than in the acidic stomach like plain aspirin does. The coating is designed to protect your stomach from direct irritation from the aspirin, and it will reduce bothersome symptoms like heartburn and stomach upset. However, it won't protect you from the stomach ulcers that aspirin can cause. This activity is caused by aspirin's effect on prostaglandins throughout the body, which is its basic action.

Taking antacids or acid-reducing H_2 blockers at the same time as enteric-coated aspirin may cause the aspirin to break down in the stomach, negating its protective effect.

Buffered

Bufferin, 325 mg

Buffering adds an antacid quality to aspirin, which will help reduce the heartburn that the drug can cause. This will provide little to no protection from possible ulcer damage in the stomach, however.

Low-Dose Aspirin

St. Joseph
Ecotrin Low Strength
Aspirin Regimen Bayer Low Strength

81-milligram aspirin is intended for long-term use for preventing cardiovascular incidents, such as heart attacks. It's sometimes called "baby aspirin."

Effervescent

Alka-Seltzer, 325 mg (original, PM), 500 mg (Morning Relief, Extra Strength)

Taking aspirin in this "highly buffered" formula can reduce stomach upset from the drug.

However, these preparations are high in sodium, so if you're on a restricted-sodium diet you should use with caution or avoid.

Combined with Caffeine

Excedrin, 250 mg (extra strength, Excedrin Migraine)
Anacin, 400 mg, 500 mg (Anacin Extra Strength)

Caffeine added to an aspirin product may help the medication act more quickly and with a lower dose. Caffeine may also help aspirin relieve some headaches by causing blood vessels in the brain to tighten, reducing blood flow.

Excedrin also contains acetaminophen, the pain reliever also found in Tylenol. Some varieties of Excedrin contain no aspirin, only acetaminophen and caffeine.

Since caffeine is a stimulant, aspirin formulations containing it may cause difficulty sleeping, nervousness, and jitters in some people.

Powdered

BC Powder, 650 mg (also contains caffeine and salicylamide, which like aspirin is a salicylate)
Goody's Headache Powder, 520 mg (also contains acetaminophen and caffeine)
Goody's Body Pain Powder, 500 mg (also contains acetaminophen)

Aspirin was originally made available in powdered form when it debuted more than one hundred years ago, and this type of aspirin has retained a following, particularly in Southern states. This powdered form may be helpful for people who can't swallow pills. It can be mixed with water or other beverages, mixed in food, or taken straight.

Chewable

Aspirin Regimen Bayer Children's Chewable Tablets, 81 mg
St. Joseph Adult Aspirin Chewable Tablets, 81 mg

This is another choice for people who have difficulty swallowing aspirin. Avoid chewing aspirin for at least seven days after oral surgery or tonsillectomy, as the product may injure tissues.

Talk to your doctor before giving aspirin to children, due to the chance of a rare but serious complication called Reye's syndrome.

Suppositories

Paddock Laboratories, Inc.
60, 120, 125, 200, 300, 325, 600, and 650 mg; 1.2 grams

Aspirin is available in suppository form for people who can't or won't take pills by mouth. This includes people who can't swallow pills, such as children or people with swallowing disorders, those who would vomit aspirin taken by mouth, or people unconscious after surgery.

Aspirin suppositories are best kept in a cool place, such as your refrigerator. However, keep them from freezing. To insert, remove the foil wrapper, moisten the suppository with cool water, lie on your side (or have the person receiving the medication do so), and insert the suppository into the rectum.

These are available at pharmacies, but you may need to ask the pharmacist to order them. Be aware that aspirin in suppository form can cause rectal irritation.

Gum

Aspergum, 227 mg

This is intended for the relief of sore throat, headache, fever, and body pain. Chew the gum for about fifteen minutes, then spit out.

Avoid aspirin gum for at least seven days after oral surgery or tonsillectomy, as the product may injure tissues.

Notes

Chapter 1. Aspirin's History and Future

1. Mann, Charles. 1991. *The Aspirin Wars.* New York: Knopf.
2. Bayer, Antony. 1998. *Clinicians' Guide to Aspirin.* London: Arnold.
3. Mueller, Richard. 1994. "History of drugs for thrombotic disease." *Circulation* 89(1):432–39.
4. Elwood, Peter. 2001. "Aspirin: past, present and future." *Clinical Medicine* 1(2):132–37.
5. Tainter, Maurice. 1969. *Aspirin in Modern Therapy.* Sterling Drug.
6. Chemical Heritage Foundation. 2001. "Coal tar" [online, cited 17 November 2004]: www.chemheritage.org/EducationalServices/pharm/glossary/coaltar.htm.
7. Vane, John. 2003. "The mechanism of action of aspirin." *Thrombosis Research* 5–6:255–58.
8. Aspirin Foundation. "100 years of aspirin" [online, cited 17 November 2004: www.aspirin-foundation.com/what/100.html.
9. Food and Drug Administration. 1999. "An aspirin a day" [online, cited 17 November 2004]: www.fda.gov/fdac/features/1999/299_asp.html.

10. Food and Drug Administration. 1999. "Healthy People 2010" [online, cited 24 November 2004]: www.healthypeople.gov/Document/HTML/uih/uih_2.htm.

11. Ayres, Stephen. 1996. *Health Care in the United States*. Chicago: American Library Association.

12. Beers, Mark. 1899. *The Merck Manual of Diagnosis and Therapy.*

13. Turnock, Bernard. 2003. *Public Health: What It Is and How It Works*. Boston: Jones & Bartlett.

14. Merson, Michael. 2000. *International Public Health*. Boston: Jones & Bartlett.

15. Centers for Disease Control and Prevention. "Fast stats" [online, cited 24 November 2004]: www.cdc.gov/nchs/fastats/Default.htm.

16. American Cancer Society. 2004. "Cancer facts and figures" [online, cited 17 November 2004]: www.cancer.org/downloads/STT/CAFF_finalPWSecured.pdf.

17. National Institutes of Health. "What makes coronary artery disease more likely?" and "Who gets angina?" [online, cited 17 November 2004]: www.nhlbi.nih.gov/health/dci/Diseases/Cad/CAD_WhoIsAtRisk.html and www.nhlbi.nih.gov/health/dci/Diseases/Angina/Angina_WhoIsAtRisk.html.

18. American Stroke Association. 2004. "About stroke" [online, cited 17 November 2004]: www.strokeassociation.org/presenter.jhtml?identifier=11402.

19. American Diabetes Association. 2002. "National diabetes fact sheet" [online, cited 18 November 2004]: www.diabetes.org/diabetes-statistics/national-diabetes-fact-sheet.jsp.

20. Food and Drug Administration. 1999. "An aspirin a day" [online, cited 18 November 2004]: www.fda.gov/fdac/features/1999/299_asp.html#other.

Chapter 2. How It Works

1. Bayer, Antony. 1998. *Clinicians' Guide to Aspirin*. London: Arnold.

2. "The Nobel Prize in physiology or medicine," 1982 [online, cited

18 November 2004]: www.nobelprize.org/medicine/laureates/1982/index.html.

3. "Adventures and excursions in bioassay: the stepping-stones to prostacyclin," 1982 [online, cited 18 November 2004]: www.nobelprize.org/medicine/laureates/1982/vane-lecture.pdf.

4. Norman, A. W. 1997. Burlington: Academic Press.

5. Crofford, Leslie. 2001. "Prostaglandin biology." *Gastroenterology Clinics of North America* 30(4):863–76.

6. McEvoy, Gerald. 2004. *AHFS Drug Information.* Bethesda: American Society of Health-System Pharmacists.

7. Lacy, Charles. 2003. *Lexi-Comp's Drug Information Handbook.* Hudson: Lexi-Comp.

8. Shannon, Margaret. 2001. *Health Professional's Drug Guide.* Upper Saddle River, N.J.: Prentice-Hall.

9. Micromedex. 2004. *USP DI Drug Information for the Health Care Professional.* Englewood: Micromedex.

10. Awtry, Eric. 2000. "Aspirin." *Circulation* 101(10):1206–18.

11. Lingappa, Vishwanath. 2000. *Physiological Medicine.* New York: McGraw-Hill.

12. Crofford, Leslie. 2001. "Prostaglandin biology." *Gastroenterology Clinics of North America* 30(4):863–76.

13. Hersh, Elliot. 2000. "Over-the-counter analgesics and antipyretics." *Clinical Therapeutics* 22(5):500–48.

14. Rudolph, Colin. 2002. *Rudolph's Pediatrics.* New York: McGraw-Hill.

15. Cryer, Byron. 2001. "Mucosal defense and repair." *Gastroenterology Clinics of North America* 30(4):877–94.

16. 2002. "Aspirin and its rivals." *Harvard Men's Health Watch* 7(5): 1–5.

17. Food and Drug Administration. 2004. "Vioxx questions and answers [online, cited 18 November 2004]: www.fda.gov/cder/drug/infopage/vioxx/vioxxQA.htm.

18. FitzGerald, Garret. 2004. "Coxibs and cardiovascular disease." *New England Journal of Medicine* (17):1709–11.

Chapter 3. Heart Health

1. Bayer, Antony. 1998. *Clinicians' Guide to Aspirin*. London: Arnold.
2. Mann, Charles. 1991. *The Aspirin Wars*. New York: Knopf.
3. Mueller, Richard, 1994. "History of drugs for thrombotic disease." *Circulation* 89(1):432–39.
4. American Heart Association. 2004. "Get with the guidelines" [online, cited 17 November 2004]: www.americanheart.org/presenter. jhtml?identifier=3013897.
5. Aspirin Foundation. "Heart attacks" [online, cited 18 November 2004]: www.aspirin.org/prof01.html.
6. National Institutes of Health. "What is angina?" [online, cited 18 November 2004]: www.nhlbi.nih.gov/health/dci/Diseases/Angina/ Angina_WhatIs.html.
7. 2002. "Physicians health study I" [online, cited 18 November 2004]: www.phs.bwh.harvard.edu/phs1.htm.
8. Eidelman, Rachel. 2003. "An update on aspirin in the primary prevention of cardiovascular disease." *Archives of Internal Medicine* 163:2006–10.
9. American Heart Association. 2004. "Aspirin in heart attack and stroke prevention" [online, cited 19 November 2004]: www. americanheart.org/presenter.jhtml?identifier=4456.
10. Phibbs, Brendan. 1997. *The Human Heart*. Philadelphia: Lippincott Williams and Wilkins.
11. American Heart Association. 2004. "Heart, how it works" [online, cited 19 November 2004]: www.americanheart.org/presenter.jhtml? identifier=4642.
12. National Institutes of Health. "What is coronary heart disease" [online, cited 18 November 2004]: www.nhlbisupport.com/chd1/ chdexp.htm.
13. American Heart Association. 2004. "What is atherosclerosis?" [online, cited 18 November 2004]: www.americanheart.org/ presenter.jhtml?identifier=228.
14. American Heart Association. 2004. "What is angina pectoris?" [online, cited 18 November 2004]: www.americanheart.org/ presenter.jhtml?identifier=4472.

15. American Heart Association. 2002. "What is a heart attack?" [online, cited 18 November 2004]: www.americanheart.org/downloadable/heart/1041881480081WhatIsaHeart%20Attack. pdf.

16. Libby, Peter. 2002. "Inflammation and atherosclerosis." *Circulation* 105(9):1135–43.

17. Verheugt, Freek. 2002. "Aspirin beyond platelet inhibition." *American Journal of Cardiology* 90:39–41.

18. American Heart Association. 2004. "Inflammation, heart disease and stroke: the role of c-reactive protein" [online, cited 18 November 2004]: www.americanheart.org/presenter.jhtml?identifier=4648.

19. Mayo Clinic. 2004. "Novel risk factors: identifying new culprits in heart disease" [online, cited 18 November 2004]: www.mayoclinic.com/invoke.cfm?id=HB00031.

20. Paoletti, Rodolfo. 2004. "Inflammation in atherosclerosis and implications for therapy." *Circulation* 109(3):20–26.

21. Serebruany, Victor. 2004. "Risk of bleeding complications with antiplatelet agents." *American Journal of Hematology* 75:40–47.

22. Hayden, Michael. 2002. "Aspirin for the primary prevention of cardiovascular events." *Annals of Internal Medicine* 136(2):161–72.

23. American Heart Association. 2004. "How does inflammation relate to heart disease and stroke risk?" [online, cited 17 November 2004]: www.americanheart.org/presenter.jhtml?identifier=4648.

24. National Institutes of Health. "Design, rationale and objectives" [online, cited 17 November 2004]: www.nhlbi.nih.gov/about/framingham/design.htm.

25. American Heart Association. 2004. "Prevention, secondary" [online, cited 17 November 2004]: www.americanheart.org/presenter.jhtml?identifier=4723.

26. CAPRIE Steering Committee. 1997. "A randomised, blinded, trial of clopidogrel versus aspirin in patients at risk of ischaemic events." *Lancet* 348(9038):1329–39.

27. Cannon, Christopher. 2002. "Effectiveness of clopidogrel versus aspirin in preventing acute myocardial infarction in patients with symptomatic atherothrombosis." *American Journal of Cardiology* 90:760–62.

28. Gaspoz, Jean-Michel. 2002. "Cost-effectiveness of aspirin, clopidogrel, or both for secondary prevention of coronary heart disease." *New England Journal of Medicine* 346(23):1800–06.

29. American Diabetes Association. "Diabetes: Heart disease and stroke" [online, cited 18 November 2004]: www.diabetes.org/diabetes-heart-disease-stroke.jsp.

30. Krein, Sarah. 2002. "Aspirin use and counseling about aspirin among patients with diabetes." *Diabetes Care* 25(6):965–70.

31. Colwell, John. 2004. "Aspirin therapy in diabetes." *Diabetes Care* 27:S72–73.

32. American Heart Association. 1997. "Aspirin as a therapeutic agent in cardiovascular disease" [online, cited 17 November 2004]: www.americanheart.org/presenter.jhtml?identifier=1760.

33. Mayo Clinic. 2004. "Heart attack signs and symptoms" [online, cited 17 November 2004]: www.mayoclinic.com/invoke.cfm?objectid=335BD208-F892-4D6A-A14CBCB0FBF85238&dsection=2.

34. Mason, Peter. 2004. "Aspirin resistance: current concepts." *Rev. Cardiovascular Medicine* 5(3):156–63.

35. American Heart Association. 2002. "Aspirin resistance increases risk of death" [online, cited 20 November 2004]: www.americanheart.org/presenter.jhtml?identifier=3001556.

36. Amerian Heart Association. 2003. "What is coronary angioplasty?" [online, cited 17 November 2004]: www.americanheart.org/downloadable/heart/1046795664928WhatIsCoronaryAngioplasty.pdf.

37. Smith, Sidney. 2001. "ACC/AHA guidelines for percutaneous coronary intervention" (revision of the 1993 PTCA guidelines). *Journal of the American College of Cardiology* 37(8):2215–38.

38. Society of Thoracic Surgeons. "Coronary artery bypass grafting surgery" [online, cited 20 November 2004]. www.sts.org/doc/3706#1.

39. American College of Cardiology/American Heart Association. 2004. "ACC/AHA guideline update for coronary artery bypass graft surgery" [online, cited 20 November 2004]: www.acc.org/clinical/guidelines/cabg/index.pdf.

40. Topol, Eric. 2004. "Failing the public health—Rofecoxib, Merck,

and the FDA." *New England Journal of Medicine* 351(17): 1707–09.

41. Topol, Eric. "Good Riddance to a Bad Drug." *New York Times,* Oct. 2, 2004.

42. FitzGerald, Garret. 2004. "Coxibs and cardiovascular disease." *New England Journal of Medicine* 351(17):1709–11.

Chapter 4. Peripheral Arterial Disease

1. Bollinger, A. 2004. "The galloping history of intermittent claudication." *Vasa* 29(4):295–99.

2. Sugar, O. 1994. "Pioneer investigator in intermittent claudication." *Spine* 19(3):346–49.

3. American Academy of Family Physicians. "What is peripheral arterial disease?" [online, cited 20 November 2004]: www.familydoctor.org/008.xml.

4. Mohler, Emile. 2003. "Peripheral arterial disease: identification and implications." *Archives of Internal Medicine* 163(19): 2306–14.

5. Federman, Daniel. 2004. "Peripheral arterial disease." *Geriatrics* 59(4):26–36.

6. "Atherosclerosis" [online, cited 18 November 2004]: www.emedicine.com/med/topic182.htm.

7. Libby, Peter. 2002. "Inflammation in atherosclerosis." *Nature* 420 (6917):868–74.

8. Lesho, Emil. 2004. "Management of peripheral arterial disease." *American Family Physician* 69:525–33.

9. Kim, Chin. 2003. "Pharmacological treatment of patients with peripheral arterial disease." *Drugs* 63(7):637–47.

10. Doyle, Jeanne. 2003. "Pharmacotherapy and behavioral intervention for peripheral arterial disease." *Reviews in Cardiovascular Medicine* 4(1):18–24.

11. National Guideline Clearinghouse. 2001. "Antithrombotic therapy in peripheral arterial occlusive disease" [online, cited 19 November 2004]: www.guideline.gov/summary/summary.aspx?doc_id=2732.

Chapter 5. Strokes

1. Bumgarner, John. 1994. *The Health of the Presidents.* Jefferson: Mcfarland & Co.
2. Centers for Disease Control and Prevention. 2004. "Stroke/ cerebrovascular disease" [online, cited 19 November 2004]: www.cdc.gov/nchs/fastats/stroke.htm.
3. American Heart Association. 2004. "New stats show heart disease still America's no. 1 killer, stroke no. 3" [online, cited 19 November 2004]: www.americanheart.org/presenter.jhtml?identifier= 3018015.
4. Bowman, James. 2003. *Strokes.* Upper Saddle River, N.J.: Prentice-Hall.
5. American Stroke Association. 2004. "Stroke risk factors" [online, cited 19 November 2004]: www.strokeassociation.org/presenter. jhtml?identifier=4716.
6. 2002. "Stroke" [online, cited 19 November 2004]: www.4woman. gov/faq/african_american.htm.
7. National Institutes of Health. 2004. "Questions and answers about stroke" [online, cited 18 November 2004]: www.ninds.nih.gov/ health_and_medical/pubs/stroke_backgrounder.htm.
8. American Heart Association. 2004. "What is atrial fibrillation?" [online, cited 18 November 2004]: www.americanheart.org/presenter. jhtml?identifier=4451.
9. American Heart Association. 2004. "What is a transient ischemic attack?" [online, cited 18 November 2004]: www.americanheart. org/presenter.jhtml?identifier=4781.
10. Berg, A. O. 2002. "Aspirin for the primary prevention of cardiovascular events." *Annals of Internal Medicine.* 136(2):157–60.
11. Guyton, Arthur. 2000. *Textbook of Medical Psychology.* Philadelphia: W. B. Saunders.
12. Davies, Andrew. 2001. *Human Physiology.* London: Churchill Livingstone.
13. Gorelick, Phillip. 2003. "North American perspective of antiplatelet agents." *Advances in Neurology* 92:281–91.

14. CAPRIE Steering Committee. 1996. "A randomised, blinded, trial of clopidogrel versus aspirin in patients at risk of ischaemic events." *Lancet* 348(9038):1329–39.

15. Mohr, J. P. 2001. "A comparison of warfarin and aspirin for the prevention of recurrent ischemic stroke." *New England Journal of Medicine* 345(20):1444–51.

16. American Stroke Association. 2004. "Learn to recognize a stroke" [online, cited 18 November 2004]: www.strokeassociation.org/presenter.jhtml?identifier=1020.

17. Hart, R. G. 2003. "Antithrombotic therapies for stroke prevention in atrial fibrillation." *Advances in Neurology* 92:249–56.

18. Rockson, Stanley. 2004. "Comparing the guidelines: anticoagulation therapy to optimize stroke prevention in patients with atrial fibrillation." *Journal of the American College of Cardiology* 43(6):929–35.

19. Mayo Clinic. "Atrial fibrillation—screening and diagnosis" [online, cited 18 November 2004]: www.mayoclinic.com/invoke.cfm ?objectid=F553CA62-FA20-4C2B-97C29F6EAF1F81EC&dsection=5.

20. American Heart Association. 2004. "How can I make my lifestyle healthier?" [online, cited 18 November 2004]: www.americanheart.org/downloadable/stroke/107523622372950-0064%20ASA%20LifestyleChgPrv.pdf.

21. National Institutes of Health. 2004. "Brain basics" [online, cited 18 November 2004]: www.ninds.nih.gov/health_and_medical/pubs/preventing_stroke.htm.

22. Texas Heart Institute. 2004. "Carotid endarterectomy" [online, cited 18 November 2004]: www.tmc.edu/thi/carotidendar.html.

23. Bhatt, D. L. 2001. "Dual antiplatelet therapy with clopidogrel and aspirin after carotid artery stenting." *Journal of Invasive Cardiology* 13(12):767–71.

24. Danesh-Meyer, Helen. 2003. "Giant cell arteritis: managing the ophthalmic medical emergency." *Clinical and Experimental Ophthalmology* 31:173–75.

Chapter 6. Alzheimer's and Dementia

1. Bick, Katherine. 1987. *The Early Story of Alzheimer's Disease*. New York: Raven Press.
2. Cheston, Richard. 1999. *Understanding Dementia*. London: Taylor & Francis.
3. National Institute on Aging. "General information" [online, cited 18 November 2004]: www.alzheimers.org/generalinfo.htm#howmany.
4. Alzheimer's Association. 2004. "Statistics about Alzheimer's disease" [online, cited 18 November 2004]: www.alz.org/AboutAD/Statistics.asp.
5. Jacques, Alan. 2000. *Understanding Dementia*. London: Churchill Livingstone.
6. National Institute of Aging. "Neurons and their jobs" [online, cited 20 November 2004]: www.alzheimers.org/unraveling/05.htm.
7. National Institutes of Health. 2004. "Brain basics" [online, cited 18 November 2004]: www.ninds.nih.gov/health_and_medical/pubs/brain_basics_know_your_brain.htm#cortex.
8. National Institutes of Health. 2004. "The life and death of a neuron" [online, cited 18 November 2004]: www.ninds.nih.gov/health_and_medical/pubs/NINDS_Neuron.htm.
9. National Library of Medicine. 2004. "MedlinePlus" [online, cited 18 November 2004]: www.nlm.nih.gov/medlineplus/ency/article/000739.htm.
10. American Academy of Family Physicians. 2002. "Dementia: what are the common signs?" [online, cited 18 November 2004]: www.familydoctor.org/662.xml.
11. National Institutes of Health. 2004. "Forgetfulness: it's not always what you think" [online, cited 18 November 2004: www.niapublications.org/engagepages/forgetfulness.asp.
12. Ho, Lap. 1999. "Regional distribution of cyclo-oxygenase-2 in the hippocampal formation in Alzheimer's disease." *Journal of Neuroscience Research* 57(3):295–303.
13. Roman, Gustavo. 2003. "Vascular dementia: distinguishing characteristics, treatment, and prevention." *Journal of the American Geriatric Society* 51:296–304.

14. Zandi, Peter. 2002. "Reduced incidence of AD with NSAID but not H2 receptor antagonists." *Neurology* 59:880–86.

15. Veld, B. A. 2002. "Pharmacologic agents associated with a preventive effect on Alzheimer's disease." *Epidemiologic Reviews* 24(2): 248–68.

16. Nilsson, Sven. 2003. "Does aspirin protect against Alzheimer's dementia?" *European Journal of Clinical Pharmacology* 59:313–19.

17. Landi, Francesco. 2003. "Non-steroidal anti-inflammatory drug (NSAID) use and Alzheimer disease in community-dwelling elderly patients." *American Journal of Geriatric Psychiatry* 11: 179–85.

18. 2004. "Alzheimer's disease anti-inflammatory prevention trial (ADAPT)" [online, cited 21 November 2004]: www.clinicaltrials. gov/show/NCT00007189.

19. Nelson, Mark. 2003. "Rationale for a trial of low-dose aspirin for the primary prevention of major adverse cardiovascular events and vascular dementia in the elderly: Aspirin in Reducing Events in the Elderly (ASPREE)." *Drugs Aging* 20(12):893–903.

20. 2004. "Alzheimer's disease" [online, cited 21 November 2004]: www. yalenewhavenhealth.org/library/healthguide/en-us/illnessconditions/ topic.asp?hwid=support/hw136828.

Chapter 7. Digestive Cancers

1. National Cancer Institute. "Harnessing apotosis to destroy cancer cells" [online, cited 18 November 2004]: www.plan.cancer.gov/ discovery.html.

2. Balkwill, Fran. 2001. "Inflammation and cancer: back to Virchow?" *Lancet* 357(9255):539–45.

3. Bertagnolli, M. M. 2003. "The potential of non-steroidal anti-inflammatory drugs (NSAIDs) for colorectal cancer prevention." *Journal of Clinical Oncology* 84(3):113–19.

4. American Cancer Society. 2004. "What are the risk factors for colorectal cancer?" [online, cited 18 November 2004]: www. cancer.org/docroot/CRI/content/CRI_2_4_2X_What_are_the_risk_ factors_for_colon_and_rectum_cancer.asp?rnav=cri.

5. Mayo Clinic. 2003. "Colon polyps" [online, cited 18 November 2004]: www.mayoclinic.com/invoke.cfm?id=DS00511.

6. Lingappa, Vishwanath. 2000. *Physiological Medicine.* New York: McGraw-Hill.

7. American Cancer Society. 2004. "How many people get colorectal cancer?" [online, cited 21 November 2004]: www.cancer.org/docroot/CRI/content/CRI_2_2_1X_How_Many_People_Get_Colorectal_Cancer.asp?sitearea=.

8. American Cancer Society. 2004. "Cancer facts and figures" [online, cited 18 November 2004]: www.cancer.org/downloads/STT/CAFF_finalPWSecured.pdf.

9. American Cancer Society. 2000. "Colorectal cancer rates higher in African Americans" [online, cited 18 November 2004]: www.cancer.org/docroot/NWS/content/NSW_1_1x_Colorectal_Cancer_Rates_Higher_in_African_Americans.asp.

10. American Cancer Society. 2004. "What is colorectal cancer?" [online, cited 18 November 2004]: www.cancer.org/docroot/CRI/content/CRI_2_4_1x_What_Is_Colon_and_Rectum_Cancer.asp?rnav=cri.

11. University of Iowa. 1998. "Colon polyps" [online, cited 18 November 2004]: www.uihealthcare.com/topics/aging/agin3367.html.

12. Mayo Clinic. 2003. "Colon polyps" [online, cited 18 November 2004]: www.mayoclinic.com/invoke.cfm?objectid=C9BB1E4C-12DB-4916-86E2CE5E70BDB744&dsection=6.

13. Crohn's and Colitis Foundation of America. 2004. "Introduction to Crohn's disease" [online, cited 18 November 2004]: www.ccfa.org/research/info/aboutcd.

14. Crohn's and Colitis Foundation of America. 2004. "Understanding colorectal cancer" [online, cited 18 November 2004]: www.ccfa.org/frameviewer/?url=/media/pdf/cancer.pdf.

15. Itzkowitz, S. H. 2004. "Colorectal cancer in inflammatory bowel disease." *American Journal of Gastroenterological and Liver Physiology* 287(1):G7–17.

16. American Cancer Society. 2002. "Oncogenes and tumor suppressor genes" [online, cited 18 November 2004]: www.cancer.

org/docroot/ETO/content/ETO_1_4x_oncogenes_and_tumor_
suppressor_genes.asp.

17. Thibodeau, Gary. 2002. *The Human Body in Health and Disease.*
St. Louis: Mosby.

18. Neighbors, Marianne. 2000. *Human Diseases.* Albany, N.Y.: Thomson Delmar.

19. American Cancer Society. 2002. "Chronic inflammation linked
to cancer" [online, cited 18 November 2004]: www.cancer.
org/docroot/NWS/content/NWS_1_1x_Chronic_Inflammtion_
Linked_to_Cancer.asp.

20. American Cancer Society. 2000. "Scientists study beginnings of
cancer formation" [online, cited 18 November 2004]: www.
cancer.org/docroot/NWS/content/NWS_1_1x_Scientists_Study_
Beginnings_of_Cancer_Formation.asp.

21. Sandler, R. S. 2003. "A randomized trial of aspirin to prevent colorectal adenomas in patients with previous colorectal cancer."
New England Journal of Medicine 348(10):883–90.

22. Chan, A. T. 2003. "A prospective study of aspirin use and the risk for
colorectal adenoma." *Annals of Internal Medicine* 140(3):157–66.

23. Sandler, R. S. 2004. "Aspirin prevention of colorectal cancer:
more or less?" *Annals of Internal Medicine* 140(3):224–25.

24. National Institutes of Health. 2002. "Barrett's esophagus" [online,
cited 18 November 2004]: www.digestive.niddk.nih.gov/ddiseases/
pubs/barretts/.

25. National Institutes of Health. 2003. "Heartburn, hiatal hernia,
and GERD" [online, cited 18 November 2004]: www.digestive.
niddk.nih.gov/ddiseases/pubs/gerd/index.htm.

26. American Cancer Society. 2002. "Esophageal cancer" [online,
cited 18 November 2004]: www.cancer.org/downloads/PRO/
EsophagealCancer.pdf.

27. Corley, D. A. 2003. "Protective association of aspirin/NSAIDs and
esophageal cancer." *Gastroenterology* 124(1):47–56.

28. Hur, Chin. 2004. "Cost-effectiveness of aspirin chemoprevention
for Barrett's esophagus." *Journal of the National Cancer Institute*
96(4):316–25.

29. American Cancer Society. 2004. "Cancer facts and figures" [online, cited 18 November 2004]: www.cancer.org/downloads/STT/CAFF_finalPWSecured.pdf.

30. Crew, K. D. 2004. "Epidemiology of upper gastrointestinal malignancies." *Seminars in Oncology* 31(4):450–64.

31. Mayo Clinic. 2003. "Stomach cancer" [online, cited 18 November 2004]: www.mayoclinic.com/invoke.cfm?objectid=4545F9D7-17A0-4275-9C296401969A8E11.

32. American Cancer Society. 2004."What are the key statistics for stomach cancer?" [online, cited 18 November 2004]: www.cancer.org/docroot/CRI/content/CRI_2_4_1X_What_are_the_key_statistics_for_stomach_cancer_40.asp?rnav=cri.

33. American Cancer Society. 2004. "What is stomach cancer?" [online, cited 18 November 2004]: www.cancer.org/docroot/CRI/content/CRI_2_4_1X_What_is_stomach_cancer_40.asp?rnav=cri.

34. Wang, W. H. 2004. "Non-steroidal anti-inflammatory drug use and the risk of gastric cancer." *Journal of the National Cancer Institute* 95(23):1784–91.

35. Thun, Michael. 2004. "Inflammation and cancer: an epidemiological perspective." *Cancer and Inflammation* 56:6–21.

Chapter 8. Breast Cancer

1. 2004. "Mammography" [online, cited 18 November 2004]: www.radiologyinfo.org/content/mammogram.htm.

2. Dullum, J. R. 2000. "Rates and correlates of discomfort associated with mammography." *Radiology* 214(2):547–52.

3. National Academies Press. 2001. "Mammography and beyond" [online, cited 18 November 2004]: www.books.nap.edu/books/0309072832/html/16.html#pagetop.

4. 2004. "History of the mammography" [online, cited 18 November 2004]: www.gehealthcare.com/inen/rad/whc/mswhhis.html.

5. American Cancer Society. 2004. "Cancer facts and figures" [online, cited 18 November 2004]: www.cancer.org/downloads/STT/CAFF_finalPWSecured.pdf.

6. American Cancer Society. 2004. "Breast cancer in men" [online, cited 18 November 2004]: www.documents.cancer.org/168.00/168.00.pdf.

7. American Cancer Society. 2004. "What is breast cancer?" [online, cited 18 November 2004]: www.cancer.org/docroot/CRI/content/CRI_2_2_1X_What_is_breast_cancer_5.asp.

8. Susan G. Komen Foundation. 2004. "Breast structure and function" [online, cited 18 November 2004]: www.komen.org/intradoc-cgi/idc_cgi_isapi.dll?IdcService=SS_GET_PAGE&ssDocName=BreastStructureAndFunction.

9. Susan G. Komen Foundation. 2004. "What is breast cancer?" [online, cited 18 November 2004]: www.komen.org/intradoc-cgi/idc_cgi_isapi.dll?IdcService=SS_GET_PAGE&ssDocName=WhatIsBreastCancer.

10. Susan G. Komen Foundation. 2004. "How hormones affect breast cancer" [online, cited 18 November 2004]: www.komen.org/stellent/groups/harvard_group/@dallas/documents/-komen_site_documents/ rfaphormones.pdf.

11. American Cancer Society. 2004. "What causes breast cancer?" [online, cited 19 November 2004]: www.cancer.org/docroot/CRI/content/CRI_2_2_2X_What_causes_breast_cancer_5.asp?rnav= cri.

12. National Institutes of Health. "Estrogen target tissues" [online, cited 18 November 2004]: www.press2.nci.nih.gov/sciencebehind/estrogen/estrogen03.htm.

13. American Cancer Society. 2000. "Estrogen and progesterone receptors" [online, cited 18 November 2004]: www.cancer.org/docroot/PED/content/PED_2_3X_Estrogen_and_Progesterone_Receptors.asp?sitearea=PED.

14. American Cancer Society. 2001. "Tamoxifen credited for improving breast cancer survival" [online, cited 18 November 2004]: www.cancer.org/docroot/NWS/content/NWS_1_1x_Tamoxifen_Credited_for_Improving_Breast_Cancer_Survival.asp.

15. Harris, Randall. 2003. "Breast cancer and nonsteroidal anti-inflammatory drugs." *Cancer Research* 63(18):6096–101.

16. Davies, G. 2002. "Cyclooxygenase-2 (COX-2), aromatase and breast cancer." *Annals of Oncology* 13(5):669–78.

17. Mayo Clinic. 2004. "Tamoxifen, aromatase inhibitors, and breast cancer" [online, cited 18 November 2004]: www.mayoclinic.com/invoke.cfm?objectid=54E3D92D-1BA1-44BA-89DBD6D1148D40A1.

18. Dubois, R. N. 2004. "Aspirin and breast cancer prevention: the estrogen connection." *JAMA* 291(20):2488–89.

19. Terry, Mary Beth. 2004. "Association of frequency and duration of aspirin use and hormone receptor status with breast cancer risk." *JAMA* (20):2433–40.

20. Johnson, Trista. 2002. "Association of aspirin and nonsteroidal anti-inflammatory drug use with breast cancer." *Cancer Epidemiology Biomarkers and Prevention* 11(12):1586–91.

21. Harris, Randall. 2003. "Breast cancer and nonsteroidal anti-inflammatory drugs." *Cancer Research* 63(18):6096–101.

22. Rodriguez, L. A. 2004. "Risk of breast cancer among users of aspirin and other anti-inflammatory drugs." *British Journal of Cancer* 91(3):525–29.

Chapter 9. Other Cancers

1. Kasum, Christine. 2003. "Non-steroidal anti-inflammatory drug use and risk of adult leukemia." *Cancer Epidemiology Biomarkers and Prevention* 12:534–37.

2. Muscat, J. E. 2003. "Risk of lung carcinoma among users of non-steroidal anti-inflammatory drugs." *Cancer* 97(7):1732–36.

3. Holick, C. N. 2003. "Aspirin use and lung cancer in men." *British Journal of Cancer* 89:1705–08.

4. Akhmedkanov, Arslan (Alan Arslan). 2002. "Aspirin and lung cancer in women." *British Journal of Cancer* 87:49–53.

5. Akhmedkanov, Arslan (Alan Arslan). 2001. "Aspirin and epithelial ovarian cancer." *Preventive Medicine* 33:682–87.

6. Hussain, T. 2003. "Cyclooxygenase-2 and prostate carcinogenesis." *Cancer Letters* 191(2):125–35.

7. Rodriguez, Luis. 2004. "Inverse association between nonsteroidal antiinflammatory drugs and prostate cancer." *Cancer Epidemiology, Biomarkers, and Prevention* 13(4):649–53.

8. Mahmud, S. 2004. "Prostate cancer and use of nonsteroidal antiinflammatory." *British Journal of Cancer* 90:93–99.

9. American Cancer Society. 2004. "Cancer facts and figures" [online, cited 18 November 2004]: www.cancer.org/downloads/STT/CAFF_finalPWSecured.pdf.

10. American Cancer Society. 2004. "Leukemia classifications" [online, cited 18 November 2004]: www.cancer.org/docroot/CRI/content/CRI_2_6X_Leukemia_Classifications_24.asp.

11. American Cancer Society. 2004. "What are the risk factors for lung cancer?" [online, cited 18 November 2004]: www.cancer.org/docroot/CRI/content/CRI_2_4_2X_What_are_the_risk_factors_for_lung_cancer_26.asp?sitearea=.

12. American Cancer Society. 2004. "What are the key statistics for lung cancer?" [online, cited 18 November 2004]: www.cancer.org/docroot/CRI/content/CRI_2_4_1X_What_are_the_key_statistics_for_lung_cancer_26.asp?sitearea=.

13. Duperron, C. 1997. "Chemopreventive efficacies of aspirin and sulindac against lung tumorigenesis in A/J mice." *Carcinogenesis* 18:1001–1006.

14. American Cancer Society. 2004. "What is lung cancer?" [online, cited 18 November 2004]: www.cancer.org/docroot/CRI/content/CRI_2_4_1X_What_is_lung_cancer_26.asp?sitearea=.

15. American Cancer Society. 2004. "What is non-Hodgkin lymphoma?" [online, cited 18 November 2004]: www.cancer.org/docroot/CRI/content/CRI_2_4_1X_What_Is_Non_Hodgkins_Lymphoma_32.asp.

16. Leukemia and Lymphoma Society. "Lymphoma" [online, cited 18 November 2004]: www.leukemia-lymphoma.org/all_page?item_id=7030.

17. Chang, E. T. 2004. "Aspirin and the risk of Hodgkin's lymphoma in a population-based case-control study." *Journal of the National Cancer Institute* 96(4):305–15.

18. Lingappa, Vishwanath. 2000. *Physiological Medicine*. New York: McGraw-Hill.

19. American Cancer Society. 2004. "Can ovarian cancer be found early?" [online, cited 18 November 2004]: www.cancer.org/docroot/ CRI/content/CRI_2_4_3X_Can_ovarian_cancer_be_found_early_ 33.asp?rnav=cri.

20. National Ovarian Cancer Coalition. "What is ovarian cancer?" [online, cited 18 November 2004]: www.ovarian.org/pages.asp? page=What%20is%20it.

21. National Institutes of Health. "Prostate cancer: causes and risk factors" [online, cited 18 November 2004]: www.nihseniorhealth. gov/prostatecancer/causeandriskfactors/02.html.

Chapter 10. Preeclampsia and In Vitro Fertilization

1. Rooks, Judith. 1999. *Midwifery and Childbirth in America*. Philadelphia: Temple University Press.

2. Mitford, Jessica. 1993. *The American Way of Birth*. New York: Plume.

3. DeCherney, Alan. 2003. *Current Obstetric and Gynecologic Diagnosis and Treatment*. Norwalk, Conn.: Appleton & Lange.

4. March of Dimes. 2004. "Pre-eclampsia" [online, cited 18 November 2004]: www.marchofdimes.com/pnhec/188_1054.asp.

5. National Institutes of Health. 2004. "Disorders of pregnancy" [online, cited 18 November 2004]: www.nichd.nih.gov/womenshealth/ disorders_of_pregnancy.cfm.

6. Caritis, S. 1998. "Low-dose aspirin to prevent preeclampsia in women at high risk." *New England Journal of Medicine* 338(11): 701–05.

7. CLASP Collaborative Group. 1994. "A randomised trial of low-dose aspirin for the prevention and treatment of pre-eclampsia among 9364 pregnant women." *Lancet* 343(8898):619–20.

8. Coomarasamy, A. 2003. "Aspirin for prevention of preeclampsia in women with historical risk factors." *Obstetrics & Gynecology* 101(6): 1319–32.

9. Branch, D. W. 2003. "Antiphospholipid syndrome." *Obstetrics and Gynecology* 101(6):1333–44.

10. Waldenstrom, U. 2004. "Low-dose aspirin in a short regimen as standard treatment in in vitro fertilization." *Fertility and Sterility* 81(6):1560–64.

11. University of Utah Health Sciences Center. 2003. "Pregnancy and childbirth" [online, cited 18 November 2004]: www.uuhsc.utah. edu/healthinfo/adult/Pregnant/stats.htm.

12. Peters, R. M. 2004. "Hypertensive disorders of pregnancy." *Journal of Obstetric, Gynecologic and Neonatal Nursing* 33(2):209–20.

13. 2004. "Antiplatelet agents for preventing pre-eclampsia and its complications." In Cochrane Database of Systematic Reviews [online database, cited 18 November 2004].

14. Food and Drug Administration. 2003. "Taking medicine while pregnant or breast-feeding" [online, cited 18 November 2004]: www.fda.gov/womens/getthefacts/pregnancy.html.

15. Micromedex. 2004. *USP DI Drug Information for the Health Care Professional.* Greenwood Village, Colo.: Thomson Micromedex.

16. Mayo Clinic. 2003. "Infertility" [online, cited 18 November 2004]: www.mayoclinic.com/invoke.cfm?objectid=5B0A05CB- 053F-4FD3-9BE06955A15A3CD9&dsection=8.

17. 2000. "Cost of IVF treatment" [online, cited 18 November 2004]: www.ivillagehealth.com/experts/fertility/qas/0,11816,166261_168 536-1,00.html.

18. Kozer, E. 2003. "Effects of aspirin consumption during pregnancy on pregnancy outcomes." *Birth Defects Research* 68(1):70–84.

19. Mayo Clinic. "Methods for optimizing your chances of pregnancy with IVF" [online, cited 18 November 2004]: www.mayoclinic. org/ivf-sct/optimizing.html.

Chapter 11. Other Conditions

1. Ganong, William. 2003. *Review of Medical Physiology.* London: Lange.

2. Carbone, Laura. 2003. "Association between bone mineral den-

sity and the use of nonsteroidal anti-inflammatory drugs and aspirin." *Journal of Bone Mineral Research* 18(10):1795–802.

3. National Osteoporosis Foundation. 2004. "Bone basics" [online, cited 18 November 2004]: www.nof.org/osteoporosis/bonehealth.htm.

4. Centers for Disease Control and Prevention. 2002. "Cytomegalovirus (CMV) infection" [online, cited 18 November 2004]: www.cdc.gov/ncidod/diseases/cmv.htm.

5. Shah, P. K. 2001. "Link between infection and atherosclerosis: who are the culprits: viruses, bacteria, both, or neither?" *Circulation* 103(1):5–6.

6. Streblow, D. N. 2001. "Do pathogens accelerate atherosclerosis?" *Journal of Nutrition* 131:2798S–804S.

7. Speir, E. 1998. "Aspirin attenuates cytomegalovirus infectivity and gene expression mediated by Cyclooxygenase-2 in coronary artery smooth muscle cells." *Circulation Research* 83:210–16.

8. National Library of Medicine. 2003. "Kawasaki disease" [online, cited 18 November 2004]: www.nlm.nih.gov/medlineplus/ency/article/000989.htm.

9. Rudolph, Colin. 2002. *Rudolph's Pediatrics.* New York: McGraw-Hill.

10. Hay, William. 2003. *Current Pediatric Diagnosis and Treatment.* Los Altos, Calif.: Lange.

11. Tierney, Lawrence. 2004. *Current Medical Diagnosis and Treatment.* Los Altos, Calif.: Lange.

12. Stuart, B. J. 2004. "Polycythemia vera." *American Family Physician* 69(9):2139–44.

13. National Library of Medicine. 2004. "Polycythemia vera" [online, cited 18 November 2004]: www.nlm.nih.gov/medlineplus/ency/article/000589.htm.

14. *Merck Manual.* "Polycythemia vera" [online, cited 18 November 2004]. www.merck.com/mmhe/sec14/ch178/ch178b.html.

15. Spivak, J. L. 2003. "Chronic myeloproliferative disorders." *American Society of Hematology Education Program Book.* Available: www.asheducationbook.org.

Chapter 12. Everyday Uses

1. Hersh, Elliot. 2000. "Over-the-counter analgesics and antipyretics." *Clinical Therapeutics* 22(5):500–48.
2. U.S. Headache Consortium. "Evidence-based guidelines for migraine headache in the primary care setting: pharmacological management of acute attacks" [online, cited 18 November 2004]: www.aan.com/professionals/practice/pdfs/gl0090.pdf.
3. Wenzel, R. G. 2003. "Over-the-counter drugs for acute migraine attacks: literature review and recommendations." *Pharmacotherapy* 23(4):494–505.
4. American Council for Headache Education. 2004. "What you should know about headache" [online, cited 18 November 2004]: www.achenet.org/understanding/.
5. National Headache Foundation. "Categories of headache" [online, cited 18 November 2004]: www.headaches.org/consumer/presskit/NHAW04/Categories%20of%20Headache.pdf.
6. Robbins, Lawrence. 2002. *Management of Headache and Headache Medications.* New York: Springer-Verlag.
7. 2004. "Headache, migraine" [online, cited 18 November 2004]: www.emedicine.com/oph/topic463.htm.
8. National Headache Foundation. "Rebound headache" [online, cited 18 November 2004]: www.headaches.org/consumer/educational modules/completeguide/other.html.
9. Arthritis Foundation. "Drug guide 2004" [online, cited 18 November 2004]: www.arthritis.org/conditions/DrugGuide/about_nsaids.asp.
10. Tierney, Lawrence. 2004. *Current Medical Diagnosis and Treatment.* Los Altos, Calif.: Lange.
11. Arthritis Foundation. 2004. "Osteoarthritis" [online, cited 18 November 2004]: www.arthritis.org/conditions/DiseaseCenter/oa.asp.
12. Arthritis Foundation. "Rheumatoid arthritis" [online, cited 18 November 2004]: www.arthritis.org/conditions/DiseaseCenter/RA/default.asp.
13. Taylor, Robert. 2003. *Family Medicine, Principles and Practice.* New York: Springer-Verlag.

14. Arthritis Foundation. "NSAIDs" [online, cited 18 November 2004]: www.arthritis.org/conditions/DrugGuide/chart_nsaids.asp.

15. McEvoy, Gerald. 2004. *AHFS Drug Information*. Bethesda: American Society of Health-System Pharmacists.

Chapter 13. Reducing the Risk of Bleeding

1. Cryer, Byron. 2001. "Mucosal defense and repair." *Gastroenterology Clinics of North America* 30(4):877–94.

2. de Abajo, F. J. 2001. "Risk of upper gastrointestinal bleeding and perforation associated with low-dose aspirin as plain and enteric-coated formulations." *BMC Clinical Pharmacology* 1(1):1.

3. Derry, S. 2000. "Risk of gastrointestinal haemorrhage with long-term use of aspirin." *British Medical Journal* 321:1183–87.

4. National Institutes of Health. 2004. "What I need to know about peptic ulcers" [online, cited 18 November 2004]: www.digestive. niddk.nih.gov/ddiseases/pubs/pepticulcers_ez/index.htm#6.

5. National Institutes of Health. 2004. "H. pylori and peptic ulcer" [online, cited 18 November 2004]: www.digestive.niddk.nih.gov/ ddiseases/pubs/hpylori/index.htm.

6. Lanas, A. 2002. "Helicobacter pylori increases the risk of upper gastrointestinal bleeding in patients taking low-dose aspirin." *Alimentary Pharmacological Therapy* 16(4):779–86.

7. Fendrick, A. Mark. 2002. "A clinician's guide to the selection of NSAID therapy." *P&T* 27(11)579–81.

8. 2004. "Treatment strategies to promote risk reduction and healing" [online, cited 18 November 2004]: www.medscape.com/ viewarticle/473972_28.

9. Micromedex. 2004. *USP DI Drug Information for the Health Care Professional*. Greenwood Village, Colo.: Thomson Micromedex.

10. 2004. "Thwarting an aspirin allergy." *Harvard Health Letter* 15(1):3.

11. Jenkins, C. 2004. "Systematic review of prevalence of aspirin induced asthma and its implications for clinical practice." *BMJ* 328 (7437):434.

12. Szczeklik, A. 2003. "Aspirin-induced asthma." *Current Reviews of Allergy and Clinical Immunology* 111(5):913–21.

13. American Stroke Association. 2004. "Stroke risk factors" [online, cited 18 November 2004]: www.strokeassociation.org/presenter. jhtml?identifier=4716.

14. National Institutes of Health. 2003. "Your guide to lowering blood pressure" [online, cited 18 November 2004]: www.nhlbi.nih.gov/ health/public/heart/hbp/hbp_low/hbp_low.pdf.

Chapter 14. Warnings

1. Micromedex. 2004. *USP DI Drug Information for the Health Care Professional.* Greenwood Village, Colo.: Thomsen Micromedex.

2. University of Maryland School of Medicine. 2001. "Aspirin" [online, cited 24 November 2004]: www.umm.edu/altmed/consdrugs/ aspirincd.html.

3. National Reye's Syndrome Foundation. 2003. "What is Reye's syndrome?" [online, cited 24 November 2004]: www.reyesyndrome.org/ what.htm.

4. National Library of Medicine. 2004. "Reye's syndrome" [online, cited 24 November 2004]: www.nlm.nih.gov/medlineplus/ency/ article/001565.htm.

5. Kamienski, Mary. 2003. "Reye's syndrome." *American Journal of Nursing* 103(7):54–57.

6. MedicinePlus. 1994. "Bismuth subsalicylate" [online, cited 24 November 2004]: www.nlm.nih.gov/medlineplus/druginfo/uspdi/ 202092.html.

Chapter 15. New Forms of Aspirin

1. 2003. "Good news about gut-friendly aspirin." *Harvard Health Letter* 28(10):7.

2. Fiorucci, S. 2003. "Gastrointestinal safety of no-aspirin (NCX-4016) in healthy human volunteers. *Gastroenterology* 124:600-607.

3. Fiorucci, S. 2004. "Co-administration of nitric oxide-aspirin (NCX-4016) and aspirin prevents platelet and monocyte activation and protects against gastric damage induced by aspirin in humans." *Journal of the American College of Cardiology* 44(3):635–41.

4. 2004. "Key products" [online, cited 18 November 2004]: www. nicox.com/pages/keyprods.html#ncx4016.

5. 2004. "Clinical pipeline" [online, cited 18 November 2004]: www.nicox.com/pages/keyprods.html#ncx1022.

Appendix: Types of Aspirin and Their Uses

Mayo Clinic. "Salicylates" [online, cited 24 November 2004]: www.mayoclinic.com/invoke.cfm?objectid=5271E812-D7eb-4f94-9659106783FD19B3.

Index